the Abs Diet for Women

the Abs Diet for Women

The Six-Week Plan to Flatten Your Belly
and Firm Up Your Body for Life

DAVID ZINCZENKO

Editor-in-Chief of

WITH TED SPIKER

www.theAbsDiet.com

For women everywhere who know
how much we love, need, and admire them:
Here's the next step to a
happier, healthier, fitter you.

Contents

Foreword

FOR THE VERY FIRST ABS DIET book, I wrote a blurb for the cover: "Finally, a diet that's focused on what you can eat, not what you can't!" Well, after several variations on the theme (*The Abs Diet Eat Right Every Time Guide*; *The Abs Diet Get Fit, Stay Fit Plan*; *The Abs Diet 6-Minute Meals for 6-Pack Abs*), I am happy to endorse this new one—*The Abs Diet for Women*. Now I can say, "Finally, a diet that addresses the unique and personal issues for women." From PMS to postpregnancy weight, the Abs Diet looks at the science behind the recommendations. Filled with realistic and practical advice, the book offers suggestions that can become second nature.

The writing style is entertaining, the information enlightening, the sidebars and facts intriguing. I know David Zinczenko has been doing his research—to find out what is important to women. *The Abs Diet for Women* specifically addresses pregnancy, breastfeeding, and losing that baby weight in a safe and effective manner. This includes a postpartum workout that is appropriate for this very sensitive time in a woman's life. There is, of course, bone health to consider, along with the reality of feeding the kids and the stress of everyday life.

Women want to know about being vegetarian, the weight-loss implications of antidepressants, and some medical issues like irritable bowel syndrome and lactose intolerance. These are all addressed in *The Abs Diet for Women*. Although the original diet does not advocate strict calorie restriction, David heard from women that calorie counting *helps* them, and so a guide to safe, effective calorie counting is now integrated into the Abs Diet for those who want it. From shopping lists to menu plans, recipes, and clearly illustrated exercises, the Abs Diet will help any woman get closer to her weight and health goals.

We know that exercise alone is not an effective way to *lose* weight, but we also know that exercise helps maintain weight loss. Exercising also seems to help keep us on track and compliant, and it enhances our self-esteem, health, and well-being. Including the Abs Diet Workout along with a great nutrition plan makes perfect sense.

There is an e-mail "joke" that floats around cyberspace and comes across my computer every now and again about how God made Adam first, for practice, and then perfected Her creation by making Eve. The original Abs Diet was good, but *The Abs Diet for Women,* well, it's just better!

—Heidi Skolnik, MS, CDN, FACSM, the *Men's Health* weight-loss coach

Introduction

YOU HAVE ABS. YES, YOU.

The Plan That Will Turn Your Fat into Muscle

WHEN YOU THINK OF ABS, you may think of Brad Pitt or Janet Jackson. You may think of magazine covers and underwear commercials. You may think of six-packs, washboards, and a belly so tight that you could bounce a diamond off it. Your cynical side may also think of airbrushing, starvation diets, and an exercise regimen so time-consuming it would violate labor laws. Abs, you assume, are reserved for athletes, for models, for bodybuilders, for trainers, for rappers, for the half-dressed "talent" on infomercials, for genetic freaks, for the liposuctioned, and for women who would classify celery as a dessert.

Your conclusion: You have a better chance of finishing the Boston Marathon barefoot than you do of getting great abs and a flat belly.

As the editor-in-chief of *Men's Health* magazine, I know that you—no matter how big, round, or droopy your belly; how many diets you've tried; or how tempting the Boston barefoot challenge sounds—can develop a flat stomach. See, I analyze health and fitness information the way brokers analyze the market. It's my job to find the fastest, best, and smartest ways for you to make tremendous gains in your most important investment: your body. So when I think about flat stomachs, the only thing I think about is this: how you can get one.

I understand the struggle. You look down, see a Jell-O mold

implanted in your stomach or on your hips or thighs, and figure that your days of having a flat belly vanished the day you graduated from high school or gave birth to Junior. But in a way, you really shouldn't think of your abdominal muscles as being extinct. Think of your flat stomach as the third cousin you met at a past family reunion. You remember seeing her, so you have a vague memory of what she looks like, but it's been so long that you really don't have a clue where to find her now. Well, even if it's been decades since you've made any kind of contact, the physiological fact remains: You have abs.

The Abs Diet is going to help you flatten your belly so you can find them.

At a time when more than 130 million Americans are overweight or obese and when weight-loss news garners as much front-page attention as celebrity scandals (well, almost as much), there's never been a more critical time to focus on your weight, your shape, and your health. I know that some critics see flat bellies as the modern American symbol of vanity, but dropping pounds, inches, and dress sizes is more than just a way to support the mirror industry.

A flat stomach—that is, abs that show—is the contemporary badge of fitness because it's the ultimate predictor of your health.

Depending on where you fall on the body-shape scale, there's a good chance you've searched for your abs before. Maybe you've failed on previous weight-loss attempts, and maybe you've yo-yoed more than kids at a toy store. I know what you've gone through; I've talked to and heard from thousands of folks—men and women alike—who have shared their weight-loss success stories with me. But I also know what you've gone through because I, too, know what it's like to feel fat.

As a latchkey kid growing up in the early '80s, I made every mistake in the book. I ate fast food instead of smart food. I played video games when I should've been playing outside. By the time I reached 14, I was carrying 212 pounds of torpid teenage tallow on my 5-foot-10 frame. I wanted to be built like a basketball player, but instead I was built like the basketball. And I paid for it with a steady bombardment of humiliation. My older brother, Eric, would invite friends to our house just to watch me eat lunch. "Don't disturb the big animal," he'd tell his friends. "It's feeding."

Like most kids, I learned my health habits from my parents, particularly my father. He was more than 100 pounds overweight for most of his adult life. Over time, he developed hypertension and diabetes, had a minor heart attack, and would have to stop at the top of a short flight of stairs just to catch his breath. A massive stroke ended his life at 52. My father died because he ignored many signals of failing health—especially the fat that padded his gut.

But I got lucky. When I graduated from high school, I joined the Naval Reserve, where the tenets of fitness were pounded into me, day after day after day. Soon after I graduated from college, I joined *Men's Health* and learned the importance of proper nutrition and—just as important—the danger of carrying around too much fat in your stomach.

Belly fat—the fat that pushes your waist out—is the most dangerous fat on your body. And it's one of the reasons why the Abs Diet emphasizes losing belly fat—because doing so means you'll live longer. Belly fat is classified as visceral fat; that means it is located behind your abdominal wall and surrounds your internal organs. Because it carries an express-lane pass to your heart and other important organs, visceral fat is the fat that can kill you. Just consider one University of Alabama–Birmingham study in which researchers used seven different measurements to determine a person's risks of cardiovascular disease. They concluded that the amount of visceral fat the subjects carried was the single best predictor of heart disease risk.

Whether you want to change your body to improve your health, your looks, your energy levels, or your sex appeal, the Abs Diet offers you a simple promise: If you follow this plan, you will transform your body so that you can accomplish each and every one of those goals. As a bonus, the Abs Diet will do something more than just enhance your life; the Abs Diet is going to save it.

And in this special edition, *The Abs Diet for Women*, you'll do more than transform your body into a lean one. You'll also learn how to make the Abs Diet principles work for you specifically—considering your lifestyle, your hormones, and the fact that many of you have to deal with the one biological factor that men don't have to consider: Your belly is stretched not only by sour cream and key lime pie but also by little runts that like to nestle in there for 9 months at a time.

When you think of all you have to gain with the Abs Diet, it becomes apparent what's wrong with most diet plans out there: They're all about losing. When you consider America's obesity epidemic, losing weight is an admirable goal. But I think there's a fundamental psychological reason why many of these diets fail: There's no motivation in losing. Americans don't like to lose. We don't like to lose board games. We don't like to lose in the market. We don't like to lose our smooth skin, our teeth, or

DIET IS A FOUR-LETTER WORD

In all honesty, I hated to even call this book a "diet" book. That's because the word *diet* has been twisted around to mean something you follow temporarily—you "go on a diet." But if you "go on" a diet, you eventually have to "go off" it. And that's why most diets are really, really bad for you.

Most diets are about eating less food or about restricting you to certain kinds of food. Most of them work in the short term because if you reduce your calorie intake, your body starts to burn itself off in order to keep itself alive. Presto, you lose weight. But here's the problem: The first thing your body does when it's short of calories is to dump the body tissue that takes the most calories to maintain.

That's muscle. So on a low-calorie diet, your body burns away muscle and tries to store fat. Sure, you'll lose weight, and you'll eventually start losing fat as well. But when you "go off" your diet, you'll start to put weight back on. And guess what kind of weight you'll gain? Pure fat. Because you've taught your body a harsh lesson: It has to be on the lookout for potential low-calorie periods in the future, so it had better store fat just in case. You've also used up valuable calorie-burning muscle, so you're likely to end up fatter than you were before your diet. That's why people who try diet after diet not only don't lose weight but also gain it.

The Abs Diet isn't a shotgun, irresponsible approach to weight management. Oh, you'll lose weight, and you'll lose it fast. But you'll lose fat, not muscle. And you'll keep that weight off for life. You'll follow the tenets of the Abs Diet for life, too, because it's about eating lots and lots of great food in smart ways. So enjoy the Abs Diet. But let's keep that little four-letter word between us, okay?

our bodies' fight against gravity. We don't like to lose anything. In a way, we don't even like losing weight because we've all been force-fed the notion that bigger is better. Instead, we're programmed to gain. We want to gain fitness. We want to gain strength. We want to add to our life, not subtract from it. We want to win—and see our results. So consider the Abs Diet a shift in the way you think about your body and about weight loss. This program concentrates on what you can gain and how you can gain it. As a result of what you'll gain from this program—abs, muscle tone, energy, better health, a great sex life (more on that later)—you'll effortlessly strip away fat from your body and change your body shape forever.

No diet plan would work without good nutrition, so that, of course, is the major focus of the Abs Diet. You'll not only learn what to eat; you'll also learn how to eat to make your body burn fat furiously, as well as how to make sure that you can control the cravings that threaten to add girth to your middle. The focus of the plan revolves around—but does not restrict you to—12 "Powerfoods" that are among the best sources of protein, fiber, and all the other ingredients and nutrients that help fight fat. When you build your diet around these foods, you will build a new body in the process. But we've taken this weight-loss plan to a whole other level. While nutrition remains a principal component of most diets, too many programs out there focus solely on how to change your eating habits—cut carbs, add cabbage soup, eat at Subway twice a day. Those programs fail to recognize a crucial component of weight control: the fact that our bodies have their own natural fat-burning mechanism . . .

Muscle.

Building just a few pounds of muscle in your body is the physiological equivalent of kicking fat out on its butt and telling it to never come back again. Muscle—in the form of lean muscle mass, not bulky, bodybuilder muscle mass—exponentially speeds up the fat-busting process: One pound of muscle requires your body to burn up to 50 extra calories a day just to maintain that muscle. Now think about what happens if you add just a few pounds of toned muscle over the course of a diet program. It'll take your body up to several hundred extra calories a day just to feed that muscle; essentially, you'll burn off an extra pound of fat every few weeks without doing a thing (and that's not even including the gains you can make by changing your diet). When you combine exercise with the foods that most promote lean muscle growth, the ones that keep you full, and the ones that give your body a well-balanced supply of nutrients, you'll be in the sweet spot, doing what this plan is all about.

You'll change the shape of your body by stripping your fat and showing off your lean muscle.

Does that mean the Abs Diet is going to make you burly, muscle-bound, or governor of California? Not at all. The Abs Diet and the accompanying Abs Diet Workout emphasize leanness and muscle tone—not big, mannish muscles.

Going back to that important investment, you can think about muscle as your compound interest. If you've ever taken a basic economics course, then you understand how compound interest works: If you invest $100 in a high-yield fund and add a little more every month, over time that investment will grow and grow to half a million dollars or more. But you'll have invested only a fraction of the money yourself. Compound interest is what allows you to make the most dramatic financial gains. It's the same concept with your body. Invest in a little additional muscle in the next 6 weeks—through eating the right foods and following a muscle-adding, fat-burning exercise plan—and you'll have invested in a lean and strong body that can last a lifetime because your new muscle will continually break down fat to stay alive.

I'm passionate about this plan because I know it works. I've seen it work, and so will you. During the course of this 6-week plan, you can lose up to 20 pounds of fat (much of it in the first couple of weeks, and from your belly first) and gain several pounds of lean muscle. But the biggest thing you'll notice is that you'll have significantly changed the shape of your body. Some of you will have even more dramatic results (see page 24 for the story of Linda Toomey, who lost 16 pounds in the first 6 weeks on the diet and cut her body fat percentage from 36 to 25). The Abs Diet includes all three components to a successful body-transforming program: nutrition, exercise, and the motivational principles to follow through. I've designed this program to make it easy to stick to, even if you've tried and failed with diets in the past. It's easy to follow because:

▶ Every component of the diet and exercise plan is quick, simple, and flexible enough so that you can easily work it into your life.

▶ Every goal is attainable.

▶ Every principle is supported by well-respected scientific research.

The Abs Diet will change the way you think about your body. It's the first plan to count not just the calories your body takes in but the calories your body burns off as well. Using the most cutting-edge nutrition and exercise research, the Abs Diet will show you how to retrain your body to burn fat faster and more efficiently—even while you sleep—and to focus your meals around the foods that inspire your body to keep those calorie-burning fires stoked. The Abs Diet isn't about counting calories (though you certainly can if that works for you); it's about making your calories count.

Throughout the book, I'll take you through the principles of the Abs Diet and show you how to follow the 6-week plan. I'll also explain the exercise program (which doesn't have to start until the 3rd week) and give you instructions on how to perform the exercises and how to make the meals. (For the time-crunched, you can cook up many of our Power-food feasts with only a blender.)

To keep you motivated, I've included the stories of real-life women who credit the Abs Diet with changing their bodies and their lives—not to mention their wardrobes.

The Abs Diet Cheat Sheet

THIS AT-A-GLANCE GUIDE summarizes the principles of the Abs Diet: the 6-week plan to flatten your belly and firm up your body for life.

SUBJECT	GUIDELINE
Number of meals	Six a day, spaced relatively evenly throughout the day. Eat snacks 2 hours before larger meals.
Portion size	While many diets center around controlling portion size, the Abs Diet is designed to be self-controlling. The high-fiber, high-protein foods you'll encounter in this book will fill you up and keep you feeling full for hours. Your body will tell you when it's time to eat—and when it's time to stop. But if you like to count calories, you can use our nutritional charts in the book to help guide you.
Nutritional ingredients to emphasize	Protein, monounsaturated and polyunsaturated fats, fiber, calcium.
Nutritional ingredients to limit	Refined carbohydrates (or carbs with high glycemic index), saturated fats, trans fats, high-fructose corn syrup.
The ABS DIET POWER 12	Base most of your meals on these 12 groups of foods. Every meal should have at least two foods from the list.
	Almonds and other nuts
	Beans and legumes
	Spinach and other green vegetables

Dairy (fat-free or low-fat milk, yogurt, cheese)

Instant oatmeal (unsweetened, unflavored)

Eggs

Turkey and other lean meats

Peanut butter

Olive oil

Whole-grain breads and cereals

Extra-protein (whey) powder

Raspberries and other berries

Secret weapons	Each of the ABS DIET POWER 12 has been chosen in part for its stealthy, healthy secret weapons—the nutrients that will help power up your natural fat burners, protect you from illness and injury, and keep you lean and fit for life!
Alcohol	Limit yourself to two or three drinks per week to maximize the benefits of the Abs Diet plan.
Ultimate Powerfood	Smoothies. The combination of the calcium and protein in milk, yogurt, and whey powder, combined with the fiber in oatmeal and fruit, makes them one of the more filling, easier options in the diet. Drink them regularly.
Cheating	One meal a week, eat anything you want.
Exercise program	Optional for the first 2 weeks. Weeks 3 through 6 incorporate a 20-minute, full-body workout 3 days a week. Emphasis is on strength training, brisk walking, and some abdominal work.
At-home workout	Gym workouts and at-home workouts are both detailed to excuse-proof your fitness plan.
Abdominal workout	At the beginning of two of your strength-training workouts. Do one exercise for each of the five different parts of your abs.

Chapter I

STRIP AWAY FAT, STRIP AWAY TROUBLE

Six Ways a Flat Belly Will Dramatically Improve How You Look, Feel, and Live

IN GYMS, PLAYING FIELDS, BEACHES, AND bedrooms across the country, our bodies are constantly being measured. And in dressing room mirrors and on bathroom scales, we're constantly measuring ourselves. But let's set aside those vanity measurements and concentrate on measuring ourselves by a different set of criteria—the number of fat cells we're carrying.

The average American has about 30 billion fat cells; each of them is filled with greasy substances called lipids. When you pump doughnuts, corn chips, and fried Snickers bars into your system, those fat cells can expand—up to 1,000 times their original size. But a fat cell can get only so big; once it reaches its physical limit, it starts to behave like a long-running sitcom. It creates spin-offs, leaving you with two or more fat cells for the price of one. Only problem: Fat cells have a no-return policy. Once you have a fat cell, you're stuck with it. So as you grow fatter and double the number of fat cells in your body, you also double the difficulty you'll have losing the lipids inside them.

Many of us tend to store fat in our bellies, and that's where the health dangers of excess weight begin. Some of us store it above the belt, while others store it below the belt. In any case, abdominal fat doesn't just sit there and do nothing; it's active. It functions like a separate

3

organ, releasing substances that can be harmful to your body. For instance, it releases free fatty acids that impair your ability to break down the hormone insulin (too much insulin in your system can lead to diabetes). Fat also secretes substances that increase your risk of heart attacks and strokes, as well as the stress hormone cortisol (high levels

FAT'S DOMINOES

Overweight people are:

▶ 50 percent more likely to develop heart disease (obese: up to 100 percent)

▶ Up to 360 percent more likely to develop diabetes (obese: up to 1,020 percent)

▶ 16 percent more likely to die of a first heart attack (obese: 49 percent)

▶ Roughly 50 percent more likely to have total cholesterol above 250 (obese: up to 122 percent)

▶ 14 percent less attractive to the opposite sex (obese: 43 percent)

▶ Likely to spend 37 percent more a year at the pharmacy (obese: 105 percent)

▶ Likely to stay 19 percent longer in the hospital (obese: 49 percent)

▶ 20 percent more likely to have asthma (obese: 50 percent)

▶ Up to 31 percent more likely to die of any cause (obese: 62 percent)

▶ 19 percent more likely to die in a car crash (obese: 37 percent)

▶ 120 percent more likely to develop stomach cancer (obese: 330 percent)

▶ Up to 90 percent more likely to develop gallstones (obese: up to 150 percent)

▶ 590 percent more likely to develop esophageal cancer (obese: 1,520 percent)

▶ 35 percent more likely to develop kidney cancer (obese: 70 percent)

▶ 14 percent more likely to have osteoarthritis (obese: 34 percent)

▶ 70 percent more likely to develop high blood pressure (obese: up to 170 percent)

of cortisol are also associated with diabetes and obesity as well as with high blood pressure). Abdominal fat bears the blame for many health problems because it resides within striking distance of your heart, liver, and other organs—pressing on them, feeding them poisons, and messing with their daily function.

Now take a look at the people with flat stomachs and six-packs. They're the icons of strength and good health. They're lean; they're strong; they look good in clothes; they look good without clothes. A defined midsection, in many ways, has defined fitness. But it also defines something else: A flat stomach is the hallmark of people in control of their bodies and, as such, in control of their health.

While some people may think that working toward a flat belly is shallower than a kiddie pool, there's nothing wrong with striving for a flat stomach or a defined midsection. Of course, defined abs make you look good—and make others feel good about the way you look, too. (In one survey, both men and women rated abs as the sexiest body part.) And for good reason: When you're in great shape, you're telling the world that you're a disciplined, motivated, confident, and healthy person—and hence a desirable partner. And sometimes a little vanity can be good for your health: In a recent Canadian study of more than 8,000 people, researchers found that over 13 years, the people with the weakest abdominal muscles had a death rate more than twice as high of those with the strongest midsections. Such research upholds the notion that flat stomachs do more than turn heads at the beach. In fact, your abdominal muscles control more of your body than you may even realize—and have just as much substance as show. In short, here are my top six reasons why flattening your belly is going to make your life better.

A Flat Belly Will Help You Live Longer

STUDY AFTER STUDY shows that the people with the largest waist sizes have the most risk of life-threatening disease. The evidence couldn't be more convincing. According to the National Institutes of Health, a waistline larger than 35 inches for women signals significant risk of heart disease and diabetes. One study in the *International Journal of Obesity* found that women should strive for waist sizes less than 31.5—as your waist grows larger, so does your risk of heart disease. Now the real scary part: A study showed that the average woman's waist size is more than 36 inches—meaning she is at an increased risk for the same health problems.

Of course, finding your abs doesn't guarantee you a get-out-of-the-hospital-free card, but studies show that by developing a strong abdominal section, you'll reduce body fat and significantly cut the risk factors

BABY, BABY, WHERE DID OUR LUNCH GO?

Your last meal didn't wind up just in your stomach. After a meal, your body begins to apportion the calories to nutrient-hungry organs, growing muscles, and, yes, your belly. Michael Jenson, MD, professor of medicine in the division of endocrinology, diabetes, and metabolism at the Mayo Clinic, calculated this breakdown of how your body processes food.

10 percent to the kidneys. Kidneys work to make sure the blood is balanced with the right amounts of water and nutrients.

5–10 percent to the heart. The heart gets most of its energy from fat, which provides more long-term energy for the hardworking heart than glucose can.

23 percent to the liver, pancreas, spleen, and adrenal glands. After the liver pulls out nutrients, it stores excess calories as glycogen.

25 percent to muscles. Muscles require a constant source of energy just to maintain their mass, so the more muscle you have, the more calories you burn.

10 percent to the brain. Glucose is brain fuel. It can't be stored long-term, which is why people often feel faint if they skip a meal.

10 percent to thermogenesis. The simple act of breaking down the food you just ate takes up one-tenth of your calories.

2–3 percent to fat cells. Your fat cells grow and eventually divide as more and more calories are deposited.

10 percent to no one knows where. Your body's a big place, and some calories go unaccounted for.

associated with many diseases, not just heart disease. For example, the incidence of cancer among obese patients is 33 percent higher than among lean ones, according to a Swedish study. The World Health Organization estimates that up to one-third of cancers of the colon, kidney, and digestive tract are caused by being overweight and inactive. A University of Minnesota study that tracked 22,000 women over 7 years found that overweight women who lost 20 or more pounds cut their risk of breast cancer by 19 percent. And having an excess of belly fat is especially dangerous. See, cancer is caused by mutations that occur in cells as they divide. Fat tissue in your abdomen spurs your body to produce hormones that prompt your cells to divide. More cell division means more opportunities for cell mutations, which means more cancer risk.

A lean waistline also heads off another of our most pressing health problems—diabetes. Currently, 13 million Americans have been diagnosed with adult-onset diabetes, and many more go undiagnosed. Fat, especially belly fat, bears the blame. There's a misconception that diabetes comes only from eating too much refined sugar, like the kind in chocolate and ice cream. But people contract diabetes after years of eating high-carbohydrate foods that are easily converted into sugar—foods like white bread, pasta, and mashed potatoes. Scarfing down a basket of bread and a bowl of pasta can do the same thing to your body that a carton of ice cream does: flood it with sugar calories. The calories you can't burn are what convert into fat cells that pad your gut and leave you with a disease that, if untreated, can lead to blindness, heart attacks, strokes, amputation, and death. And that, my friend, can really ruin your day. But you can control a lot of this; a study tracking 1,400 diabetic people for 9 years found that just trying to lose weight could cut diabetes-related death risk by up to 30 percent.

Upper-body obesity is also the most significant risk factor for obstructive sleep apnea, a condition in which the soft tissue in the back of your throat collapses during sleep, blocking your airway. When that happens, your brain signals you to wake up and start breathing again. As you nod off once more, the same thing happens, and it can continue hundreds of times during the night—making you chronically groggy and unable to get the rest your body needs. (You won't remember waking up over and over again; you'll just wonder why 8 hours of sleep left you dragging.) Fat's role is that it can impede muscles that inflate and ventilate the lungs, forcing you to work harder to get enough air. When Australian researchers studied 313 patients with severe obesity, they found that 62 percent of the people with a waist circumference of 49 inches or more had a serious sleep disturbance and that 28 percent of obese patients with smaller waists (less than 49 inches) had sleep problems.

Being overweight also puts you at risk for a lot of other conditions that rob you of a good night's rest, including gastroesophageal reflux and asthma. A 3-year French study of 67,229 women found that being overweight doubled the risk of asthma. And women who gained about 20 pounds from the time they started menstruating to the time they reached adulthood had 66 percent higher risk. All of this can create an ugly cycle: Abdominal fat leads to poor sleep. Poor sleep means you drag through your day. Sluggish and tired, your body craves some quick energy, so you snack on some high-calorie junk food. That extra junk food leads to more abdominal fat, which leads to . . . well, you get the picture.

I could fill this whole book with evidence, but I'm going to boil it down to one sentence: A smaller waist equals fewer health risks.

A Flat Belly Will Improve Your Sex Life

WOMEN CLAIM THE GREATEST sex organ is the brain; men say it's approximately 3 feet due south. So let's say we split the geographic difference and focus on what's really central to a good sex life.

For one, strong abdominal and lower-back muscles give you stamina and strength to try new positions (or stay steady in old ones), so that sex is as pleasurable as it should be. But even more important, a smaller waistline means that women will be better equipped in another important area—bloodflow.

Artery-clogging cheeseburgers don't discriminate, so when you're overweight, the gunk that gums up the blood vessels leading to your heart and brain also gums up the vessels that lead to your genitals. Plaque forms on the inside of your arteries, narrowing the passageways that blood must follow—meaning that blood has trouble making it to the pelvic area. Decreased flow of blood in the pelvic area in women can lead to decreased lubrication, sensitivity, and sexual pleasure.

At least one study of more than 200 women showed that by increasing bloodflow to the genital area of women, you could increase lubrication, sensitivity, arousal, and sensation to the area. Though the results are preliminary, it does suggest that clear faucets can play a role in sexual satisfaction.

A Flat Belly Will Keep You Safe from Harm

IN SCHOOL, YOU were taught the story of Mrs. O'Leary's cow and how, with one awkward misstep, the lumbering bovine knocked over an oil lamp that started the Great Chicago Fire and burned much of that toddlin' town to the ground. That tragedy happened at a time when most urban housing was still built with wood. Today, such a disaster is unthinkable—and not just because we don't let cows into the living room anymore. It's unthinkable because the infrastructure of today's cities is built with steel—steel that stands up to fire, earthquakes, and hurricanes.

Think of your midsection as your body's infrastructure. You don't want a core made of dry, brittle wood or straw. You want one made of solid steel, one that will give you a layer of protection that belly fat never could.

Consider a US Army study that linked powerful abdominal muscles to injury prevention. After giving 120 artillery soldiers the standard army fitness test of situps, pushups, and a 2-mile run, researchers tracked their lower-body injuries (such as lower-back pain and Achilles tendinitis) during a year of field training. The 29 soldiers who cranked out the most situps (73 in 2 minutes) were five times less likely to suffer lower-body injuries than the 31 who barely notched 50. But that's not the most striking element. Those who performed well in the pushups and 2-mile run enjoyed no such protection—suggesting that upper-body strength and cardiovascular endurance had little effect on keeping bodies sound. It was abdominal strength that offered the protection. Unlike any other muscles in your body, a strong core affects the functioning of the entire body. Whether you ski, do yard work, or carry the kids away from the candy aisle, your abs are the most essential muscles for keeping you from injury. The stronger they are, the stronger—and safer—you are.

A Flat Belly Will Strengthen Your Back

I HAD A FRIEND who threw out his back maybe two or three times a year. He always did it in the simplest way—sleeping a little awkwardly or getting out of a chair too quickly. One time, he pulled it out reaching into the backseat of his car to get something his young daughter had dropped. The pain once stabbed him so badly that he collapsed to the ground while he was standing at a urinal. (Go ahead. Imagine that.) His problem wasn't that he had a bad back; it was that he had weak abs.

ABS DIET SUCCESS STORY

"I FOUND MY INNER ATHLETE"

Name: Rebecca Carr

Age: 29

Height: 5'1½"

Starting Weight: 148

Current Weight: 118

Starting Waist Size: 32¾"

Current Waist Size: 26½"

Starting Dress Size: 10

Current Dress Size: 4

Rebecca Carr always felt that she was a little bit over a healthy weight.

"Growing up, I saw people who were into fitness and health and eating right, and I always thought that they were doing something right in life. I said, 'Hey, that's how I want to live.' I always wanted to be that person," she says.

If he had trained them regularly, he could've kept himself from being one of the millions of people who suffer from back pain every year. And yes, he started the Abs Diet Workout, and within weeks his back pain virtually disappeared.

Because most back pain is related to weak muscles in your trunk, maintaining a strong midsection can help resolve many back issues. The muscles that crisscross your midsection don't function in isolation; they weave through your torso like a spiderweb, even attaching to your spine. When your abdominal muscles are weak, the muscles in your butt (your glutes) and along the backs of your legs (your hamstrings) have to compensate for the work your abs should be doing. The effect, besides promoting bad company morale for the muscles picking up the slack, is that it destabilizes the spine and eventually leads to back pain and strain—or even more serious back problems.

One morning, Carr and her husband were watching TV and heard the Abs Diet being mentioned on the morning news.

"Something just clicked in my head," she says. "It's what I believe in and it matches who I am, and it made sense. I bought the only copy of the book that was on the shelf at Borders and read it cover to cover."

Carr made adjustments to her diet, limiting her desserts and fried foods to the point where the onetime dessertaholic doesn't even miss them. (The weekly cheat meal that the Abs Diet allows keeps her in check: "If I want a burger and fries, I tell myself I can have it on the weekend if I want, but by the time the weekend comes, my interest is gone.")

Carr is never hungry, and she packs her daily meals the night before to help her manage eating during stressful days. Besides having improved skin and energy levels, Carr has also been inspired to push herself deeper into the world of fitness—she has completed 5-K and 10-K races, and now she's training for a half-marathon. "At 29 years old, I found my inner athlete," she says.

Now Carr's parents tell her that she's a different person—how motivating she is that she has such a healthy outlook. Carr's husband and father have both lost weight on the Abs Diet, having been motivated by her success.

"It doesn't feel like a diet," she says. "It feels like living."

A Flat Belly Will Help You Win

IF YOU RUN, bike, play naked Twister, or do any sport that requires movement, your essential muscle group isn't your legs or arms. It's your core—the muscles in your torso and hips. Developing core strength gives you power to perform. It fortifies the muscles around your whole midsection and trains them to provide the right amount of support when you need it. So if you're weak off the serve, strong abs will improve it. If you also play sports where you run a lot, whether it's tennis or tag, abs can improve your game tremendously. That's because speed is really about accelerating and decelerating. How fast can you go from a stopped position at one baseline to stopping at the other baseline? Your legs don't control that; your abs do. When researchers studied what muscles were the first to engage in these types of sports movements, they found that the abs fired first. The stronger they are, the faster you'll get to the ball.

A Flat Belly Will Limit Your Aches and Pains

AS YOU AGE, it's common to experience some joint pain—most likely in your knees and hips, but maybe around your feet and ankles, too. The source of that pain might not be weak joints; it might be weak abs—especially if you do any kind of exercise, from serious tennis playing to every morning walking. When you're doing any type of athletic activity, your abdominal muscles help stabilize your body during start-and-stop movements, like changing direction on the tennis court or in kickboxing class. If you have weak abdominal muscles, your joints absorb all the force from those movements. It's kind of like trampoline physics. Jump in the center, and the mat will absorb your weight and bounce you back in the air. Jump toward the side of the trampoline, where the mat meets the frame, and you'll bust the springs. Your body is sort of like a trampoline, with your abs as the center of the mat and your joints as the supports that hold the mat to the frame. If your abs are strong enough to absorb some shock, you'll function well. If they're not, the force puts far more pressure on your joints than they were built to withstand.

Similar protection benefits extend to people who aren't athletes, too. One Dutch study of nearly 6,000 people found that those with larger waist sizes were more likely to have heel pain and develop carpal tunnel syndrome, a painful hand and wrist condition. One study even found that 70 percent of people with carpal tunnel syndrome were either overweight or obese.

• • •

These are all great reasons to pursue the Abs Diet. But the best reason is this: The program is an easy, sacrifice-free plan that will let you eat the foods you want and keep you looking and feeling better day after day. It's designed to help you lose weight in the easiest possible ways: by recalibrating your body's internal fat-burning furnace; by focusing on the foods that trigger your body to start shedding flab; and by rebuilding you into a lean, mean, fat-burning machine.

THE ABS DIET
START-UP KIT

THIS SIMPLE SHOPPING LIST WILL give you everything you need to dive right into the Abs Diet and the Abs Diet Workout.

Buy Once

Blender	Ground flax-seed, 1 pint	Multivitamins, such as Centrum, 1 jar

Basic Shopping List—The ABS DIET POWER 12 and Related Foods

Almonds, slivered or whole

Beans of choice

Spinach, fresh or frozen

Dairy (fat-free or low-fat milk and vanilla yogurt)

Instant oatmeal (unsweetened, unflavored)

Eggs

Turkey, sliced

Peanut butter, all-natural (no added sugar)

Olive oil

Whole-grain breads and cereals

Extra-protein (whey) powder, vanilla and chocolate, 1 quart containers

Raspberries, fresh and frozen

Plus:

Black beans

Blueberries, frozen

Canned tuna

Cannellini beans

Chicken breast

Craisins (dried, sweetened cranberries)

Garbanzo beans

Grapefruit

Green vegetables of choice

Italian salad greens

Lean ground beef

Long-grain rice

Mixed greens

Pecans

Pine nuts

Roasted cashews and peanuts, unsalted

Shrimp, frozen

Strawberries, fresh or frozen

Trout, smoked salmon, or other lean fish of choice

Whole-wheat pasta

**Shopping List–Ingredients for Recipes
(see recipes for individual amounts)**

Avocado

Baby carrots

Balsamic and red wine vinegars

Bananas

Barbecue sauce

Basil

Beef jerky

Brown rice

Canadian bacon

Canned chicken stock

Canned mandarin orange slices

Canned peeled tomatoes

Canned pumpkin

Cantaloupe

Carnation Instant Breakfast packets

Cayenne pepper

Celery

Chili powder

Chives

Chocolate syrup

Cilantro

Cinnamon

Corn, frozen

Cornmeal

Cucumber

Curry powder

Dijon mustard

Dried chili mix

Fat-free mayonnaise

Flat bread

Flour

French green beans

Fresh ginger

Garlic

Green and red bell peppers

Guacamole

Housin sauce

Honey

Honeydew melon

Honey-wheat English muffins

Instant grits

Italian-seasoned bread crumbs

Italian seasoning

Jalapeño peppers

Ketchup

Lean sirloin steak

Lean sliced roast beef

Lemons and limes

Lemon juice concentrate, frozen

Low-fat balsamic vinaigrette, ranch, and

Thousand Island salad dressings

Low-fat ice cream (vanilla and butter pecan)

Low-fat Italian salad dressing packet

Maple syrup

Mexican-style tomatoes

Mint, fresh or dried

Mushrooms

Navy beans

Onions, green, red, and white

Onion soup mix

Orange juice

Oranges

Oregano

Paprika

Parsley

Peanut oil

Pork chops, boneless

Prosciutto

Red pepper flakes

Reduced-fat cheese (American, blue cheese, Cheddar, cottage, cream, feta, mozzarella, ricotta, Swiss)

Raisin bread

Raisins

Red and Granny Smith apples

Reduced-sodium soy sauce

Roasted red peppers

Romaine lettuce

Rosemary

Rye bread

Salsa

Saltine crackers or bread crumbs

Sauerkraut

Spaghetti sauce

Stir-fry sauce

Sweet corn

Tabasco sauce

Tomatoes

Tomato sauce

Tortilla chips

Trans fat–free margarine

Turkey bacon

Turkey sausage

Watermelon

Whole-wheat pitas

Whole-wheat toaster waffles

Whole-wheat tortillas

Worcestershire sauce

**For At-Home Exercise
(a gym should have all necessary equipment)**

Exercise mat (optional)	One or two pairs of medium-weight dumb-bells (5 to 25 pounds for someone with some experi-ence lifting weights; lighter for beginners)	Swiss ball (optional but recommended)
Flat bench (optional but recommended)	Running shoes	

Chapter 2

WHY THE ABS DIET? AND WHY NOW?

Shocking New Scientific Breakthroughs in Nutrition

THE ABS DIET IS A SIMPLE PLAN built around 12 nutrient-packed foods that, when moved to the head of your dietary table, will give you all the vitamins, minerals, and fiber you need for optimum health while triggering lean muscle growth and firing up your body's natural fat burners. I'll tell you more about these foods in an upcoming chapter, but here's a quick overview. (Tell me this isn't a meal plan you can stick to!)

Almonds and other nuts

Beans and legumes

Spinach and other green vegetables

Dairy (fat-free or low-fat milk, yogurt, cheese)

Instant oatmeal (unsweetened, unflavored)

Eggs

Turkey and other lean meats

Peanut butter

Olive oil

Whole-grain breads and cereals

Extra-protein (whey) powder

Raspberries and other berries

12!

I've chosen these foods both for their nutritional content and their simplicity. That's why I based the Abs Diet on common foods that are easy to prepare and enjoy. The way I see it, most other diet plans are too complicated and invite failure in three major ways.

1. **They reduce calories too severely.** With a strict—or drastic—calorie reduction, you may lose weight at first, but you're left hungry. When you're hungry, you've increased the chances that you'll gorge at some point during the day. When you gorge, you feel as if you failed, then feel guilty for failing, then drop off the plan and resume your chocolate-for-breakfast habits. With the Abs Diet, however, you'll never go hungry—in fact, you'll find yourself eating much more often than you do now: six times a day!

2. **They restrict too many foods.** It would be easy to build a plan that didn't include pasta, pizza, or savory bruschetta. But if

ABS DIET SUCCESS STORY

"YOU'RE GETTING WHAT WOMEN DIE FOR"

Name: Rhonda Hauser

Age: 38

Height: 5'8"

Weight: 140ish

Starting Body: Soft

Current Body: Strong

Built with a tall, lanky runner's body, Rhonda Hauser has never been one to care much about scales or taking measurements of herself. But she has been in and out of gyms for years, she's had a couple trainers, and she's gone to nutritionists because she cares about her body. But she also had a problem: Turns out she was overtraining and undereating (mostly eating kashi cereal and protein shakes). She wasn't overweight, but she didn't have the body she wanted.

"I saw the Abs Diet and thought it was really targeted for me," she says. "It reminded me that you have to eat, and you need foods with protein to build muscle, the internal fat burner."

I did that, you'd ditch the plan the first time you drove past your favorite Italian restaurant. Even though changing your eating habits is a fundamental part of this program, I think there's a greater chance you'll stick to the plan if you don't have to give up everything you like. It's normal to have steaks off the grill, Mom's pie at the holidays, a glass of wine or beer after work. If you deprive yourself of every food that tastes good, there's not much incentive for even the most motivated person to stick to the plan for longer than a few weeks. The Abs Diet is about eating the foods you enjoy—and indulging yourself when need be.

3. They don't take into account lifestyle. If we all had a chef to prepare our meals—or even more than a few minutes to do it ourselves—losing weight would be much simpler. But when was the last time you had 2 hours to prepare a meal? We're all busy

---

Hauser integrated more Powerfoods into her diet and exchanged her mostly running regimen for the Abs Diet circuit workouts.

"When I started doing circuits, my body took on its own transformation," says Hauser, who got more definition in her arms and shoulders. "After a couple of weeks, people in the gym were looking at me and asking if I was training for an Ironman. I started feeling stronger, and my muscles were developing."

After 6 weeks, Hauser says, her pants started to feel a little weird. She hoped that she wasn't gaining weight from doing the exercises, so she asked her girlfriends if they could tell what was going on. "My glutes started to lift up and tighten. My friends said, 'You're getting what women die for.' I call it the hubba heinie—a little round rump roast."

While Hauser still doesn't use a scale, she knows that her body has experienced a major change.

"The cool thing about it is that it gives me direction, and it's something I believe in," Hauser says. "Anything you believe in and consistently do is going to get you results. I carry this book around with me like it's my bible."

We eat in restaurants. We order in. We hit drive-thrus. We hustle food on the table to satisfy the needs of our families and to save as much energy as possible. Yes, we wish we had time to tally fat-gram totals; measure every ounce of food; or prepare elaborate, good-for-you dishes. But the reality is that most of us won't, no matter how much weight we need to lose. We have commitments to jobs and families, and we spend so much time doing everything from commuting to paying the bills and taking care of the kids that a mango-shrimp masterpiece hardly tops the priority list. The Abs Diet is what you need: a low-maintenance program with low-maintenance foods and even lower-maintenance recipes.

For these reasons, many of today's most popular diets offer only short-term weight loss and long-term weight gain.

As I said in the introduction to this book, most diets are about losing—and Americans don't like to be losers. The Abs Diet is about gaining. The Abs Diet is based on the simple notion that your body is a living, breathing, calorie-burning machine and that by keeping your body's fat furnace constantly stoked with lots and lots of the right foods—and this is important—at the right time, you can teach it to start burning off your belly in no time. In fact, this diet can help you burn up to 12 pounds of fat—from your belly first—in 2 weeks or less. And just look at what you'll gain in return.

You'll gain meals. Americans have huge appetites. We hunger for success, we hunger for freedom, and yeah, we hunger for food. Traditional calorie- or food-restricting diets run counter to this uniquely American appetite. They leave us hungry, miserable, and one Twinkie away from a total couch collapse. But not the Abs Diet. You will eat on this program—and eat often. In fact, you'll be refueling constantly, and with every delicious meal or snack, you'll be stoking your body's natural fat burners. Imagine that: Every time you eat, you help your body lose weight and turn flab into abs.

You'll gain some tone. With the Abs Diet and the Abs Diet Workout, eating the right foods means you'll be growing more muscle. With added muscle, you'll lose more fat. This program converts the food you eat into muscle. The more lean muscle mass you have, the more energy it takes to fuel it—meaning that calories go toward sustaining your muscles rather than being converted to fat. In fact, research shows that adding lean muscle mass acts as a built-in fat burner. Again, for every pound of muscle you gain, your resting metabolic rate goes up as much as 50 calories a day. The strength-training component can put several pounds of muscle onto your body. You won't beef up like a bodybuilder, but you will build enough muscle to shrink and tighten your belly—and, depending on your starting point, show off your abs. When you add exercise into the mix, you can think of it as a simple equation.

MORE FOOD + MORE MUSCLE = LESS FLAB

Now, consider the alternative.

LESS FOOD + LESS MUSCLE = MORE FLAB

Isn't it incredible that most diets focus on the "less food" equation? And isn't it time we changed that? (Sure, some studies have shown that you'll live longer on a superrestrictive diet of less than 1,400 calories a day. But given how such a plan would make you feel, you probably wouldn't want to.)

You'll gain freedom. Most diets deprive you of something—whether it's carbs, fat, or fun. (Can I have a blue-cheese bacon burger, hold the bun? No thanks.) In this plan, you will not feel deprived. You'll stay full. You'll eat crunchy food. You'll eat sweet food. You'll eat protein, carbs, and fat. In fact, there's even one meal during the week when you can eat anything you want. Anything. During the bulk of the week, you'll focus on foods that will charge your metabolism and control your temptations, but you'll also have the freedom and flexibility to stray just enough to keep you satisfied without ruining all the work you've already put in.

You'll gain time. On some diets, it seems like it would take less time to raise a farm of chickens and wait for the eggs to drop than it would take to plan and cook the recipes they tout. On this diet, all of the meals and recipes are low maintenance. For planning purposes, all I want you to do is take this program 2 days at a time. Because mindless noshing is the nation's number one diet buster, your best defense is to plot out a simple strategy for how and what you're going to eat each day. Every night, take 5 minutes to sketch out what and when you'll eat the next day, and you'll have deflated temptation and gained control. After reading the principles, you'll see that the Abs Diet establishes a new paradigm for weight control. Simply:

MORE FOOD + MORE MUSCLE = LESS FLAB

Chapter 3

BURN FAT DAY AND NIGHT

How Metabolism Shapes Your Body— And How You Can Change Yours

IN CHAPTER 2, I DISCUSSED HOW MOST popular diets are designed to offer only short-term weight loss and how following these programs sets you up not only to regain the weight you initially shed but also to actually gain even more fat in the long run. Most diets, in fact, are not long-term fat-loss plans but long-term fat-gain plans. The Abs Diet is different: It's a program that helps you rev up your body's natural fat burners and keep them revved for life.

As harmful as most diet crazes may be, diets alone aren't to blame for the obesity epidemic in America. In fact, there's plenty of blame to go around: fast food, funnel cakes, stress, sedentary lifestyles, supersizing, all-you-can-eat buffets, the demise of physical education classes, free refills, couches, movie theater popcorn, you name it. We're a society of overeaters who often hold desk jobs and would lobby to make the Bloomin' Onion its own food group. But in the battle of weight control, these are the easy targets. Instead, I'd argue, one of the reasons we keep getting fatter is that we put our faith in two things that are supposed to help us lose weight. These weight loss "double agents" reap praise for their contributions to good health, but they've also done their part in skewing the way we think about weight loss. The two culprits I blame for our obesity epidemic: nutritional labels and exercise machines.

Is Calorie Counting Right for You?

BEFORE YOU BUST A BUTTON, hear me out. Labels and machines both have their appropriate uses (the former for the simple knowledge of the vitamins, minerals, and ingredients in your food; the latter for getting people off their duffs and exercising). My beef with labels and machines is not what they do per se but the myth they perpetuate. Through their function, they feed into a way of thinking about weight loss that actually makes it harder to control weight. They've turned us into a community of heavies who worship at the altar of one seemingly omnipotent number: the calorie.

With every food you eat and with every workout you finish, you look at how many calories come in and how many calories go out. It's the turnstile theory of weight loss: If you exercise away more than you take

ABS DIET SUCCESS STORY

"I NEEDED SOMETHING THAT WAS EASY"

Name: Linda Toomey

Age: 35

Height: 5'4"

Starting weight: 145

6 weeks later: 129

When Linda Toomey had her fourth baby, she knew that she had to get the weight off. She had kept 20 pounds on from her third baby and wanted to act quickly because she knew the longer she waited, the harder it would be. At 145 pounds and with four children under the age of 6, she knew that her own health—and belly—might take a backseat to everything else going on in her life. "I'm the queen of excuses," she says.

Toomey also knew that she needed as much energy as possible—especially considering she wasn't getting a full night's sleep anyway, caring for a newborn.

"At night, I expected to be tired," she says. "But I was tired 2 hours after I woke up."

in, then you'll lose weight. Experts tell us that a pound of fat contains roughly 3,500 calories, so if you simply delete 500 calories from your daily meals, increase your daily exercise by 500 calories, or some combination thereof, you'll lose a pound of fat a week. That sounds great in theory, but in real life, the whole concept of calorie management is more likely to make you lose heart than lose weight. You hump it on the stairclimber for 30 minutes and sweat like a guest on *The O'Reilly Factor*. When you see the final readout—"Workout Completed; 300 Calories Burned!"—you feel like you've just chipped away at your belly and gotten closer to your goal. That is, until you reach for a nighttime snack and see that a serving and a half of raisin bran also equals 300 calories. What took 30 minutes to burn takes 30 seconds to dust off during *Desperate Housewives*. It's a psychological diet killer.

Of course, there's nothing wrong with using nutritional labels to

---

Toomey's goals: Get her body back, have more energy, and strengthen her back to be able to meet the demands of carrying larger-than-average children.

"I tried other diets, but being so crazy and busy, I didn't have a lot of time for exercise or food preparation. I needed something that was easy and fast to prepare," Toomey says.

She found it in the Abs Diet.

"It's not really a diet," she says. "It's a lifelong eating plan. I think knowing that you can eat carbs and don't have to resist cravings was one of the key factors. The eating plan was extremely easy to follow, and the whole family could enjoy the meals. I didn't have to prepare different foods for myself."

Toomey also included the 20-minute exercise plan and strengthened her abdominals and lower back to the point where she has no problem lifting her children.

In 6 weeks, she dropped 16 pounds and went from 36 percent body fat to 25. And she also went from a size 14 dress to size 6.

"I'm hoping it motivates a lot of women," Toomey says. "In the past, after I was pregnant, the waist was extremely hard for me. I might have lost inches from everywhere else, but the waist was my real difficult area. It's amazing how it progressed in a short time."

track what you eat or as a deterrent to stay away from high-calorie foods in the first place. In fact, many women feel like they need calorie counting to help them stay within optimal daily targets, and that's okay—as long as you keep calories in perspective. It's better to focus on what's happening inside your body during the rest of your day—when you're working, sleeping, making love, or just sitting still right now reading this book. Right this very instant, your body is either gaining fat or losing fat. The Abs Diet will train your body to lose fat while you're sitting still because the Abs Diet focuses on something other diet plans miss: your metabolism.

What Is "Metabolism"?

METABOLISM IS THE RATE at which your body burns its way through calories just to keep itself alive—to keep your heart beating, your lungs breathing, your blood pumping, and your mind fantasizing about the Caribbean while crunching year-end accounting figures or telling Timmy to go to a time-out. Your body is burning calories all the time, even while you're reading this sentence. The average woman burns about 10 calories per pound of body weight every day.

There are three main types of calorie burn that happen throughout your day. Understand how they work, and you'll understand exactly why the Abs Diet is going to turn your body into a fat-burning machine.

Calorie burn #1: The thermic effect of eating. Between 10 and 30 percent of the calories you burn each day get burned by the simple act of digesting your food. Now that's pretty cool—satisfying your food cravings actually makes you burn away calories. But not all foods are created equal: Your body uses more calories to digest protein (about 25 calories burned for every 100 calories consumed) than it does to digest fats and carbohydrates (10 to 15 calories burned for every 100 calories consumed). That's why the Abs Diet concentrates on lean, healthy proteins. Eat more of them in a sensible way, and you'll burn more calories.

Calorie burn #2: Exercise and movement. Another 10 to 15 percent of your calorie burn comes from moving your muscles, whether you're pressing weights overhead, running to catch the bus, or just twiddling your thumbs. Simply turning the pages of this book will burn calories.

Calorie burn #3: Basal metabolism. This one's the biggie. Your basal, or resting, metabolism refers to the calories you're burning when you're doing nothing at all. Sleeping, watching TV, sitting through yet another mind-numbing presentation on corporate profit-and-loss statements—you're burning calories all the while. In fact, between 60 and 80 percent of your daily calories are burned up just doing nothing. That's because your body is constantly in motion: Your heart is beating, your lungs are breathing, and your cells are dividing all the time, even when you sleep.

Add up the percentages, and you'll see that the majority of your daily calorie burn comes from physiological functions that you don't even think about—the thermic effect of eating and your basal metabolism. While exercise is important, you need to realize that the calories you burn off during exercise aren't that important. Let me repeat that: Exercise is important, but the calories you burn off during exercise aren't important. That's why the exercise program we outline in the Abs Diet is designed to alter your basal metabolism, turning your downtime into fat-burning time. And it's why the food choices we outline for you are designed to maximize the number of calories you burn simply by eating and digesting. I want you to forget about the calories you're burning during those 30 minutes in the gym and concentrate on the calories you're burning the other 23½ hours a day.

In effect, the Abs Diet is going to change your body into a fat-frying dynamo by several means.

Changing the Way You Exercise

HAVE YOU EVER seen a gym at rush hour? Everyone hovers around the treadmills, elliptical trainers, and stationary bikes. Signs warn you of 20-minute maximums so that the next sweat seeker can have his or her turn. It seems like everyone wants a cardiovascular, aerobic workout. The more you sweat, the more calories you burn, the more weight you lose, right? In a way, yes, the headphone-and-Lycra set is right. Cardiovascular exercise—steady-state endurance exercises, like running, biking, and swimming—burns a lot of calories. In fact, it often burns more than other forms of exercise like strength training or trendier workouts like yoga or Pilates. But when it comes to weight control, aerobic exercise is more overrated than the fall TV lineup. Why? For one reason: Aerobic exercise builds little (if any) muscle, and muscle is the key component of a speedy metabolism. Muscle eats fat; again, add 1 pound of muscle, and your body burns up to an additional 50 calories a day just to keep that muscle alive. Add 6 pounds of muscle, and suddenly you're burning up to 300 more calories each day just by sitting still.

Here's the problem with low-intensity aerobic exercise. Just like a car can't run without gas or a kite can't fly without wind, a body can't function without food. It's the fuel that helps you run, lift, and have sex. Generally, during exercise, your body calls upon glycogen (the stored form of carbohydrate in muscles and the liver), fat, and in some cases protein. When you're doing low-intensity aerobic exercise like jogging, your body primarily uses fat and glycogen (carbohydrates) for fuel. When it continues at longer periods (20 minutes or more), your body drifts into depletion: You exhaust your first-tier energy sources (your glycogen stores), and your body hunts around for the easiest source of energy it can find—protein. Your body actually begins to eat up muscle tissue, converting the protein stored in your muscles into energy you need to keep going. Once your body reaches that plateau, it burns up 5 to 6 grams of protein for every 30 minutes of ongoing exercise. (That's roughly the amount of protein you'll find in a hard-cooked egg.) By burning protein, you're not only missing an opportunity to burn fat but also losing all-important and powerful muscle. So aerobic exercise actually decreases muscle mass. Decreased muscle mass ultimately slows down your metabolism, making it easier for you to gain weight.

Now here's an even more shocking fact: When early studies compared cardiovascular exercise to weight training, researchers learned that people who engaged in aerobic activities burned more calories during exercise than those who tossed around iron. You'd assume, then, that aerobic exercise was the way to go. But that's not the end of the story.

It turns out that while lifters didn't burn as many calories during their workouts as the folks who ran or biked, they burned far more calories over the course of the next several hours. This phenomenon is known as the afterburn—the additional calories your body burns off in the hours and days after a workout. When researchers looked at the metabolic increases after exercise, they found that the increased metabolic effect of aerobics lasted only 30 to 60 minutes. The effects of weight training lasted as long as 48 hours. That's 48 hours during which the body was burning additional fat. Over the long term, both groups lost weight, but those who practiced strength training lost only fat, while the runners and bikers lost muscle mass as well. The message: Aerobic exercise essentially burns only at the time of the workout. Strength training burns calories long after you leave the gym, while you sleep, and maybe all the way until your next workout. Plus, the extra muscle you build through strength training means that in the long term, your body keeps burning calories at rest just to keep that new muscle alive.

That raises a question. What aspect of strength training creates the long afterburn? Most likely, it's the process of muscle repair. Weight lifting causes your muscle tissues to break down and rebuild themselves at a higher rate than normal. (Muscles are always breaking down and rebuilding; strength training simply accelerates the process.) That breakdown and rebuilding takes a lot of energy and could be what accounts for the long period of calorie burning. In fact, a Finnish study found that protein synthesis (the process that builds bigger muscles) increases 21 percent 3 hours after a workout.

The good news is that you don't have to lift like a Russian shot-putter to see the results. A recent Ohio University study found that a short but hard workout had the same effect as longer workouts. Using a circuit of three exercises in a row for 31 minutes, the subjects were still burning more calories than normal 38 hours after the workout. (The Abs Diet Workout is designed along similar principles to mimic these results.)

As I said earlier, building muscle increases your metabolism so much that you burn up to 50 calories per day per pound of muscle you have.

(continued on page 34)

WHAT THE HECK IS . . . HIGH BLOOD PRESSURE?

You know high blood pressure is bad, but you probably have a little trouble getting your head around the whole concept of how "blood pressure" works. *Can't we just let a little of the blood out and lower the pressure?* you might wonder. If only it were so easy.

When most people think of blood pressure, they think in terms of a garden hose: too much pressure and the hose bursts, unless you open the valve. But that model is too simple. It helps instead to think of your circulatory system as more like the Erie Canal—a series of locks and gates that help move blood around to where it's needed. See, gravity works on your blood just like it works on the rest of your body: It wants to pull everything downward. So imagine yourself hopping out of bed tomorrow morning and standing up. Gravity wants to take all that blood that's distributed throughout your body and pull it down into your feet. You, on the other hand, would like that blood to pump to your brain, where it can help you figure out where the hell your keys are.

On cue, arteries in the lower body constrict while the heart dramatically increases output. The instant result: Blood pressure rises, and blood flows to the brain. Ahh, there they are—in the dog's water dish, right where you left them.

It's an ingenious system, but one that's incredibly easy to throw out of whack. When you pack on extra padding around your stomach, your heart pumps harder to force blood into all that new fatty tissue. When you nosh on potato chips and other high-sodium foods, your body retains water in order to dilute the excess sodium, increasing overall blood volume. When you line your arteries with plaque from too many fatty meals, pressure increases as the same amount of blood has to squeeze through newly narrowed vessels. When you let the pressures of the day haunt you into the night, your brain pumps out stress hormones that keep your body in a perpetual state of fight-or-flight anxiousness, also forcing your heart to pump harder. High-salt, high-fat diets and an excess of stress all combine to create a dangerous situation.

Much to the dismay of Quentin Tarantino fans, letting out some blood won't relieve the pressure. Your heart is still pumping, and your blood vessels are still dilating and contracting to make sure the blood goes where it's needed. When the pressure remains high for years on end, thin-walled vessels in the brain can burst under extreme pressure; brain cells die as a result in what's known as a hemorrhagic stroke. Or hypertension can cause plaque buildup in one of the brain's arteries, eventually cutting off bloodflow. (High blood pressure damages smooth artery walls, creating anchor points for plaque to latch on to.) Kidney failure or a heart attack can also follow from dangerous plaque accumulations.

Then there's the plain old wear and tear that high blood pressure causes on your ticker. Over time, the extra work brought on by high blood pressure causes the walls of the heart to stiffen and thicken. The heart becomes a less efficient pump, unable to push out as much blood as it takes in. Blood backs up, the heart gives out, and the coroner scribbles "congestive heart failure" on your chart.

Ideally, your blood pressure should be 120/80 or lower. What do those numbers mean? The top number, called the systolic pressure, is the pressure generated when the heart beats. The bottom number is the diastolic pressure, the pressure on your blood vessels when the heart is resting between beats. Higher readings are broken out into three categories.

▶ **Prehypertensive: 120–139 systolic/80–89 diastolic.** Prehypertensives should start worrying now about their blood pressure, concentrating on diet and exercise tips like those found in the Abs Diet. You may not see the flashing lights in your mirror right now, but your radar detector just went off. Time to slow down.

▶ **Stage I hypertensive: 140–159 systolic/90–99 diastolic.** For people who fall in this range, drug therapy is usually recommended in addition to lifestyle changes. Your risk of heart attack or stroke is elevated, and you need to be under a doctor's care.

▶ **Stage II hypertensive: 160 or greater systolic/100 or greater diastolic.** Advanced drug therapy is often a must for people at this level, who face a serious risk of being maimed or killed by their condition.

So, two questions: Do you know what your blood pressure is? If not, are you freaked out enough by now to start taking care of it? Fortunately, the Abs Diet Powerfoods can help by cutting down on the bad fats in your diet and increasing the good ones—and by slashing away some of those extra pounds. So can the Abs Diet Workout, as well as a few stress-reduction techniques. (To find out how you can help manage your stress level, see Chapter 12) In the meantime, try attacking the problem with some of these simple tips.

Make it a low-sodium V8. Make that two 5.5-ounce cans: 11 ounces of V8 contains nearly 1,240 milligrams (mg) of potassium. In a study published in the *Journal of Human Hypertension*, researchers found that prehypertensive patients who added more potassium to their diets lowered their systolic pressure by 2.5 points and their diastolic by 1.6 points. Potassium helps sweep excess sodium from the circulatory system, causing the blood vessels

(continued)

WHAT THE HECK IS . . . HIGH BLOOD PRESSURE? *(CONT.)*

to dilate. What makes V8 better than a banana (another good source of potassium)? V8 also contains lycopene and lutein, two phytochemicals that have their own blood pressure–lowering properties.

Cut out the cold cuts. One slice of ham contains 240 milligrams of sodium, more salt than you'll find on the outside of two pretzel rods. The point: Lose the lunchmeat, and lower your blood pressure. A recent study found that prehypertensive people who reduced their daily sodium consumption from 3,300 to 1,500 milligrams knocked nearly 6 points off their systolic blood pressure and close to 3 off their diastolic. If you want to have your hoagie and eat it, too, at least switch to the Boars Head line of low-sodium meats— ham, turkey, roast beef—and leave the pickle on your plate (833 milligrams of sodium). Another rule of thumb: If a food comes canned or jarred, it's probably a salt mine.

Go two rounds and out. Make the second drink of the night your last call for alcohol. In a landmark study published in the *New England Journal of Medicine*, researchers found that one or two drinks a day actually decreased blood pressure slightly. Three drinks or more a day, however, elevated blood pressure by an average of 10 points systolic and 4 diastolic. The type of alcohol doesn't matter. Heck, order a screwdriver: Orange juice is one of the best sources of blood pressure–lowering potassium.

Drink more tea. An American Heart Association study found that people who drank 2 cups of tea a day were 25 percent less likely to die of heart disease than those who rarely touched the stuff. The reason: Flavonoids in the tea not only improve blood vessels' ability to relax but also thin the blood, reducing clotting.

Top your toast. Black currant jelly is a good source of quercetin, an antioxidant that Finnish researchers believe may improve heart health by preventing the buildup of the free radicals that can damage arterial walls and allow plaque to penetrate.

Have a Mac(intosh) attack. People who frequently eat apples have a 20 percent lower risk of developing heart disease than those who eat apples less often.

Eat fresh berries. Raspberries, strawberries, and blueberries are all loaded with salicylic acid—the same heart disease fighter found in aspirin.

Order the tuna. Omega-3 fats in tuna and other fish as well as flaxseed help strengthen heart muscle, lower blood pressure, prevent clotting, and reduce levels of potentially deadly inflammation in the body.

Squeeze a grapefruit. One grapefruit a day can reduce arterial narrowing by 46 percent, lower your bad cholesterol level by more than 10 percent, and help drop your blood pressure by more than 5 points.

Feast on potassium. Slice a banana (487 milligrams) on your cereal, then bake two small sweet potatoes (612 milligrams) or cook up some spinach (1 cup has 839 milligrams) for dinner. All are loaded with potassium. Studies show that not getting at least 2,000 milligrams of potassium daily can set you up for high blood pressure. Other good sources of potassium include raisins (1 cup, 1,086 milligrams), tomatoes (1 cup sauce, 811 milligrams), lima beans (1 cup, 955 milligrams), and papayas (one has 781 milligrams of the mineral).

Buy calcium-fortified OJ. Increasing the calcium in your diet can lower your blood pressure. You'll derive a benefit from the vitamin C as well. According to research from England, people with the most vitamin C in their bloodstreams are 40 percent less likely to die of heart disease.

Snack on pumpkin seeds. One ounce of seeds contains 151 milligrams of magnesium, more than a third of your recommended daily intake. Magnesium deficiencies have been linked to most risk factors for heart disease, including high blood pressure, elevated cholesterol levels, and increased buildup of plaque in the arteries. Other great sources: halibut (170 milligrams in 7 ounces of fish), brown rice (1 cup, 84 milligrams), chickpeas (1 cup, 79 milligrams), cashews (1 ounce, 74 milligrams), and artichokes (one gives you 72 milligrams).

Change your oil. Researchers in India found that people who replaced the corn and vegetable oils in their kitchens with monounsaturated fats (olive oil or, in this case, sesame seed oil) lowered their blood pressure by more than 30 points in just 60 days without making any other changes in their diets.

Cut down on mindless candy snacking. A compound in licorice root has been shown to spike blood pressure—especially in people who eat a lot of black licorice. Fruit-flavored licorice, however, doesn't contain the compound.

The more muscle you have, the easier it is for you to lose fat. That's why one of the components of the plan includes an exercise program that will help you add the muscle you need to burn fat and reshape your body. And it also points to one of the reasons why you should deemphasize cardiovascular, aerobic exercise if you want to lose fat: because it depletes your body's store of fat-burning muscle.

Now, before you start thinking I'm some sort of antiaerobics fanatic, let me clarify a few things: I run almost daily, and I've even completed the New York City Marathon. Aerobic exercise burns calories, helps control stress, and improves your cardiovascular fitness. It also helps lower blood pressure and improve your cholesterol profile. If your choice is aerobic exercise or no exercise, for Pete's sake, get out there and run. But when it comes to long-term weight management, I'll take gym iron over road rubber any day.

Changing the Way You Eat

FEW THINGS IN American society have failed more often than diets (with the exception of your office's copy machine). I think there's an explanation for the high failure rate. For one, many diets have revolved around low-fat menus. I'll discuss fat in a later chapter, but one of the problems with low-fat diets is that they can suppress the manufacture of testosterone, the hormone that contributes to the growth of muscle and the burning of fat. When testosterone levels are low, your body stores fat like squirrels store nuts. Many diets also fail because they don't take advantage of the single most powerful nutrient for building muscle and increasing your metabolism: protein.

Protein—in proportion with foods from other groups—works in two primary ways. First, eating more protein cranks up the thermic effect of digestion by as much as one-third. Second, protein is also the nutrient that builds calorie-consuming muscle. In effect, you get a double burn— while you're digesting food and later, as it helps build muscle. In the Abs Diet, you'll emphasize protein for these very reasons, but you'll also emphasize the most powerful sources of protein. A Danish study published in the *American Journal of Clinical Nutrition* took a group of people and gave them diets that were high in protein from either pork or soy. They found that people on the diet higher in animal protein burned 2 percent more calories during a 24-hour period than those on the soy protein diet, despite the fact that they ate slightly less food. That's 34 calories a day if you're eating a 1,700-calorie diet. In other words, if you want to burn calories, tenderloin is better than tofu.

Changing the Way You Think about the Word *Diet*

HERE'S A TYPICAL diet scenario: You nibble on a piece of toast for breakfast and some baby carrots for lunch, and you figure that puts you well ahead of the calorie-counting game. By dinner, though, you've got so many onion rings jammed into your mouth that you look like Dizzy Gillespie. If you're so restricted in what you can eat, you'll eventually act like a rebellious teen and break the rules. While most diets say "no" more than a toddler with a plate of spinach, the Abs Diet gives you options. Most diets are about restricting. This one is about fueling.

For years—or maybe for all your life—you've probably had one notion about what dieting needs to be. Restrict your foods, eat like a supermodel, sweat on the treadmill, and you'll lose fat. In reality, those could be the very reasons why you couldn't lose weight. It's why you gained back what you lost. It's the reason why your speedboat metabolism may have geared down to that of an anchored barge. It's why you don't see much progress when you try new weight-loss programs. And it's why the only real recipe many diet plans offer is a recipe for pecan-encrusted failure. What the Abs Diet will do is reprogram your circuitry. You'll stop thinking about every calorie and start thinking about how best to burn calories. Once you master that, your body will be equipped with all the tools it needs to strip away fat—and show off your belly.

Chapter 4

HOW THE ABS DIET WORKS
What Your Last Meal Is Doing
to Your Body Right Now

IN THE CRUDEST FORM, THE WAY IN WHICH food travels through your body seems simple. There's one way in and one way out, and anything left behind snowballs into a mound of fat on your stomach, over your hips, on the backs of your arms, around your thighs, or under your chin. In reality, the travel patterns of your breakfast, lunch, and dinner flow more like a Los Angeles interstate system than anything else. You've got the traffic jams (clogged arteries) and the occasional drive-by shootings (indigestion), but you also have a complex network of roads that shuttle nutrients to and from vital organs and tissues. Your ability to lose weight and gain a little muscle largely depends on how and when you fuel your body to work in that system.

In the previous chapter, I showed how the key to effective weight management is concentrating on your body's calorie burn—not on how effectively you burn calories while exercising but on how effectively you burn calories when you're not exercising. Additionally, I explained a little about how the foods you eat can affect your body's daily calorie burn. Before I explain the how-tos of the Abs Diet, you should know the most important substances and nutrients that affect the way your body processes food.

Protein: The Most Valuable Nutrient

IN JUST ABOUT every area of life, few things are as admired as versatility—a mom who can shoot a basketball as well as she can cook, a dad who can change the oil and make a mean marinara sauce, a corporate president who can also fix the computers, a quarterback who runs as well as he throws, a singer who can dance as well as she can lip-synch. In your body, protein is the most versatile player on your nutrient team. It comes in many forms and does so many things well—all without a multimillion-dollar contract.

▶ Protein builds the framework of your body, including muscles, organs, bones, and connective tissues.

▶ In the form of enzymes, it helps your body digest food.

▶ As a hormone, it tells your body when to use food as energy and when to store it as fat.

▶ It transports oxygen through your blood to your muscles and organs.

▶ As an antibody, it protects you from illness when viruses and bacteria attack.

So protein is critical for helping your body function at optimum levels. But we've made protein the foundation of the Abs Diet for four other crucial reasons.

1. It tastes good. Sliced smoked turkey. Roasted pork loin. Steamed lobster. Peanut butter. The Abs Diet is built around the foods you crave, so it's a program you're not going to have to stick to; it's a program you're going to want to stick to.

2. It burns calories even as you're indulging in it. Food contains energy in the form of chemical bonds, but your body can't use them in that form. Your body has to break down the food and extract energy from that chemical bond; that process of extracting energy itself requires energy, so your body's burning more calories to do it. That's the thermic effect of eating, as I explained in chapter 3, and protein pushes the thermic effect into high gear. It takes almost two times more energy to break down protein than it does to break down carbohydrates. So when you feed your body a greater amount of protein, your body automatically burns more calories throughout the day. When Arizona State University researchers compared the benefits of a high-protein diet with those of a high-carbohydrate diet, they found that people who ate a high-protein diet burned more than twice as many calories in the hours after their meals as those eating predominantly carbs.

3. It keeps you feeling satisfied. Research has shown that if you base your meals around protein, you'll feel fuller faster. Consider one study in the *European Journal of Clinical Nutrition*. Subjects downed one type of four different kinds of shakes—60 percent protein, 60 percent carbohydrate, 60 percent fat, or a mixture with equal amounts of all three. Then they were offered lunch. The subjects who had either the high-protein or mixed-nutrient shakes ate the least for lunch. Their shakes contained the same number of calories, but the protein made them feel fuller and therefore they ate less at lunchtime.

4. It builds muscle and keeps your body burning fat all day. Remember, muscle burns fat. When you lift and lower weights, you create microscopic tears in your muscles. To repair the tears, protein acts like the Red Cross. Your body parachutes in new protein to assess the damage and repair the muscle. Proteins fortify the original cell structure by building new muscle fibers.

This whole process through which proteins make new muscle fibers after a workout can last anywhere from 24 to 48 hours. So if you lift weights 3 days a week—triggering proteins to rush in and repair your muscles—your body essentially stays in muscle-building, and thus fat-burning, mode every day.

As you know, protein comes in many forms—such as turkey, beef, fish, nuts, and tofu. You want to concentrate on the proteins that best help build your muscles. Research has shown that animal protein builds muscle better than soy or vegetable protein does. So poultry, fish, and lean cuts of beef or pork are better choices than tofu or other soy-based products (though they are viable options, if you're a vegetarian). If you're the kind of person who likes to count, you'll want to shoot for about 1 gram of protein per pound of body weight per day—that's roughly the amount of protein your body can use every day. For a 130-pound woman, that's 130 grams of protein a day, which would break down into something like this:

3 eggs (18 grams)

2 cups of 1 percent milk (16 grams)

1 cup of cottage cheese (28 grams)

2⅓ ounces of peanuts (16 grams)

8 ounces of chicken breast (54 grams)

Combine those four reasons—an easy and delicious eating plan, greater calorie burn, less calorie intake, and more fat-burning muscle—and you can easily see how a high-protein diet translates into weight loss. In a Danish study, researchers put 65 subjects on a 12 percent protein diet, a 25 percent protein diet, or no diet (the control group). In the first two groups, the same percentage of calories—about 30 percent—came from fat. While the low-protein dieters lost an average of more than 11 pounds, the high-protein subjects lost an average of 20 pounds and ate fewer calories than the low-protein group.

The more amazing statistic wasn't how much they lost but where they lost it: The high-protein dieters also lost twice as much abdominal fat. One reason may be that a high-protein diet helps your body control its levels of cortisol, a stress hormone that causes fat to converge in the abdominal region.

Fat: Underrated, Understand?

WHEN YOU THINK of fat, you probably think of foods that have a lot of fat—or people who do. After a few years with some extra pounds, the only thing you know about fat is that you're tired of it and want to get rid of it forever. But it's probably one of your body's most misunderstood dietary nutrients, stemming from a widely held but misguided belief that fat should take much of the blame for our obesity epidemic.

In the 1980s, the US government released nutritional guidelines that essentially said we should base our diets on potatoes, rice, cereal, and pasta and minimize the foods with a lot of fat and protein. That gave way to the idea that fat makes you fat. And that gave way to a new breed of diets that said if you limit the fat in what you eat, you'll limit the fat that exercises squatter's rights on your belly. But that line of thinking didn't hold out when researchers tried to find links between low-fat diets and obesity. In 1998, for example, two prominent obesity researchers estimated that if you took only 10 percent of your calories from fat, you'd lose 16 grams of fat a day—a loss of 50 pounds in a year. But when a Harvard epidemiologist, Walter Willett, tried to find evidence that this occurred, he couldn't find any link between people who lost weight and the fact that they were on a low-fat diet. In fact, in some studies lasting a year or more, groups of people showed weight gains on low-fat diets. Willett speculated that there was a mechanism responsible for this: When the body is on a low-fat diet for a long period, it stops losing weight.

Part of the reason our bodies rebel against low-fat diets is that we need fat. For instance, fat plays a vital role in the delivery of vitamins A, D, E, and K, nutrients stored in fatty tissue and the liver until your body needs them. Fat also helps produce testosterone, which helps trigger muscle growth. And fat, like protein, helps keep you satisfied and controls your appetite. In fact, if we've learned anything about weight loss over the past several years, it's that reducing your fat intake doesn't necessarily do a darn thing to decrease your body fat. One small study, for instance, compared a high-carbohydrate diet and a high-fat diet. The researchers found that the group with the high-fat diet experienced less muscle loss than the other group. The researchers theorized that muscle protein was being spared by the higher-fat diet because fatty acids, more so than carbs, were being harnessed and used for energy.

The truth is that reasonable amounts of fat can actually help you lose weight. In a study from the *International Journal of Obesity*, researchers at Boston's Brigham and Women's Hospital and Harvard Medical School put 101 overweight people on either a low-fat diet (fat was 20 percent of the total calories) or a moderate-fat diet (35 percent of calories) and followed them for 18 months. Both groups lost weight at first, but after a year and a half, the moderate-fat group had lost an average of 9 pounds per person, whereas the low-fat dieters had gained 6 pounds. The results suggest that a healthy amount of fat is a factor in keeping your weight under control.

Here's a primer on the fats in your life.

Trans fat: BAD. More and more, you're seeing trans fat listed on food labels. Though it's in more than 40,000 packaged foods, it's so bad for you that food manufacturers have fought for years to keep it off ingredient labels. In 2003, the US Food and Drug Administration finally adopted regulations requiring manufacturers to include trans fat content on their packaging. The regulations have been phased in over the past few years. It still helps to be a smart food consumer in order to spot where the danger lies.

Trans fats were invented by grocery manufacturers in the 1950s as a way of appealing to our natural cravings for fatty foods. But there's nothing natural about trans fats. They're cholesterol-raising, heart-weakening, diabetes-causing, belly-building chemicals that, for the most part, didn't even exist until the middle of the last century, and some studies have linked them to an estimated 30,000 premature deaths in this country every year. In one Harvard study, researchers found that getting just 3 percent of your daily calories from trans fats increased your risk of heart disease by 50 percent. Three percent of your daily calories equals about 7 grams of trans fats; that's roughly the amount in a single order of fries. Americans eat an average of between 3 and 10 grams of trans fats every day.

To understand what trans fats are, picture a bottle of vegetable oil and a stick of margarine. At room temperature, the vegetable oil is a liquid, the margarine a solid. Now, if you baked cookies using vegetable oil, they'd be pretty greasy. And who would want to buy a cookie swimming in oil? So to create cookies—and cakes, nachos, chips, pies, muffins, doughnuts, waffles, and many, many other foods we consume daily—manufacturers heat the oil to very high temperatures and infuse it with hydrogen. That hydrogen bonds with the oil to create an entirely new form of fat—trans fat—that stays solid at room temperature. Vegetable oil becomes margarine. And now foods that might normally be healthy—but maybe not as tasty—become fat bombs.

Because these trans fats don't exist in nature, your body has a hell of a time processing them. Once consumed, trans fats are free to cause all sorts of mischief inside you. They raise the number of LDL (bad) cholesterol particles in your bloodstream and lower your HDL (good) cholesterol. They also raise blood levels of other lipoproteins; the more lipoproteins you have in your bloodstream, the greater your risk of heart disease. Increased consumption of trans fats has also been linked to increased risk of diabetes and cancer.

Yet trans fats are added to a shocking number of foods. They appear on food labels as partially hydrogenated oil—usually vegetable or palm oil. Go look in your pantry and freezer right now, and you won't believe how many foods include them. Crackers. Popcorn. Cookies. Fish sticks. Cheese spreads. Candy bars. Frozen waffles. Stuffing. Even foods you might assume are healthy—like bran muffins, cereals, and nondairy creamers—are often loaded with trans fats. And because they hide in foods that look like they're low in fat, such as Wheat Thins, these fats are making you unhealthy without your even knowing it.

Take control of your trans fat intake. Check the ingredient labels on all the packaged foods you buy, and if you see partially hydrogenated oil on the label, consider finding an alternative. Even foods that seem bad for you can have healthy versions: McCains shoestring french fries, Ruffles Natural reduced-fat chips, Wheatables reduced-fat crackers, and Dove dark chocolate bars are just a few of the "bad for you" snacks that are actually free of trans fats. And remember—the higher up on the ingredients list partially hydrogenated oil is, the worse the food is for you. You might not be able to avoid trans fats entirely, but you can choose foods with a minimal amount of the stuff.

The other way to avoid trans fats is to avoid ordering fried foods.

Because trans fats spoil less easily than natural fats and are easier to ship and store, almost all fried commercial foods are now fried in trans fats rather than natural oils. Fish and chips, tortillas, fried chicken—all of them are packed with belly-building trans fats. Order food baked or broiled whenever possible. And avoid fast-food joints, where nearly every food option is loaded with trans fats; drive-thru restaurants ought to come complete with drive-thru cardiology clinics.

AVOID

Margarine

Fried foods

Commercially manufactured baked goods

Any food with partially hydrogenated oil on its list of ingredients

Saturated fat: BAD. Saturated fats are naturally occurring fats found in meat and dairy products. The problem with saturated fats is that when they enter your body, they tend to do the same thing they did when they were in a pig's or cow's body: Rather than be burned for energy, they're more likely to be stored as fat in your flanks, in your ribs, even—ugh—in your loins. In fact, they seem to have more of a "storage effect" than other fats. A study from Johns Hopkins University suggests that the amount of saturated fat in your diet may be directly proportional to the amount of fat surrounding your abdominal muscles. Researchers analyzed the diets of 84 people and performed an MRI on each of them to measure fat. Those whose diets included the highest rates of saturated fat also had the most abdominal fat. Saturated fats also raise cholesterol levels, so they increase your risk for heart disease and some types of cancer.

I don't want you to eliminate saturated fats entirely; they're found in most animal products, and those food products are important to the Abs Diet for other reasons (the calcium in dairy products, the protein in meat). But I do want you to consume the low-fat and leaner versions of meat and dairy products. You want the nutritional benefit from one part of the food without high amounts of saturated fat.

AVOID

Fatty cuts of red meat

Whole-milk dairy products

Polyunsaturated fats: GOOD. There are two types of polyunsaturated fats: omega-3s and omega-6s. You've probably heard of omega-3 fatty acids. They're the fats found in fish, and a diet high in omega-3s has been shown to help protect the heart from cardiovascular disease. That's plenty enough reason to include seafood in your diet. But new evidence suggests that this type of fat can actually help you control your weight. In one study, subjects who took in 6 grams a day of fish oil supplements burned more fat during the course of a day than those who went without. Researchers suspect that a diet high in

SEAFOOD WITH THE HIGHEST OMEGA-3 CONTENT

All data are for 3-ounce servings (except for sardines, which is for 3¾ ounces). Aim for a total of 2.5 grams (g) of omega-3s per day.

TYPE OF FISH	OMEGA-3 CONTENT (G)	PREPARED
Shad	3.7	Baked
Sardines	2.4	Water-packed can
Mackerel	1.9	Broiled
Sablefish	1.9	Broiled
Salmon	1.6	Poached
Tuna	1.5	Grilled
Oysters	1.4	Boiled
Trout	1.2	Broiled
Shark	1.1	Grilled
Swordfish	1.1	Grilled
Tuna	0.07	9-oz water-packed can

omega-3s actually alters the body's metabolism and spurs it to burn fat more efficiently.

Now, you can take fish oil supplements if you want, but you'll miss the muscle-building protein benefits of real fish. The fish with the highest levels of omega-3s are the fish you probably enjoy the most already— salmon and tuna, to name two. (To see where your favorite fish falls in the omega-3 sweepstakes, see the chart on page 44.) In addition to being packed with heart-healthy, fat-burning omega-3s, fish is also a great source of lean, muscle-building protein.

There's another amazing, secret Powerfood that bodybuilders know about but you may have never even heard of: flaxseed. Flax is a seldom-used grain that's loaded with omega-3s as well as cholesterol-busting fiber. You'll find flaxseed and flaxseed oil in most health food stores. Grab it! I keep ground flaxseed in the fridge, and I toss it on breakfast cereals, into smoothies, and on top of ice cream. It's got a mild nutty flavor you'll like. It crushes cholesterol with its omega-3s, it adds artery-scouring fiber to your diet, and it might just be your best weapon against fat.

Omega-6 fatty acids also help lower bad cholesterol and raise good cholesterol. They're found in vegetable oils, meat, eggs, and dairy products. They're so common to so many foods, in fact, that only those of you currently shipwrecked on deserted islands living off flotsam and jetsam need worry about not getting enough in your diet.

EAT MORE

Fish

Flaxseed and flaxseed oil

Monounsaturated fats: GOOD. Monounsaturated fats are found in nuts, olives, peanuts, avocados, and olive and canola oils. Like omega-3s, these fats help reduce cholesterol levels and protect against heart disease, but they also help you burn fat; in one study, researchers found that the body burns more fat in the 5 hours following a meal high in monos than after a meal rich in saturated fats.

Monounsaturated fats will not only lower your cholesterol and help you burn off your belly but also help you eat less. Penn State researchers found that people who ate mashed potatoes prepared with oil high in monounsaturated fats like olive oil felt fuller longer than when they ate taters cooked with polyunsaturated fats like vegetable oil.

Carbohydrates: A Bad Rap

WITH THE BEATINGS that carbohydrates have taken over the past few years, it's a wonder that bread isn't protected by the Endangered Species Act. Everywhere I look, I see people eating burgers without buns, ordering spaghetti and meatballs—hold the spaghetti—or bragging about their all-bacon-all-the-time diet. While it's clear that protein and fat have tremendous nutritional benefits, it's unfair—and unhealthy—to kick carbohydrates off the dietary island.

INSULIN: THE TWO-FACED HORMONE

The hormone insulin is like your pack-rat grandmother: It likes to store stuff. The only problem is that it's also as schizophrenic as old Uncle Judd. Sometimes it makes your muscles grow; sometimes it makes your fat cells grow.

Different foods create different insulin responses. Foods that have high–glycemic index rankings (including white bread, most cereals, grapes, and bananas) dump a lot of sugar into your bloodstream soon after you eat them, causing insulin levels to spike. In this case, insulin works quickly to turn that blood sugar into fat.

Some foods, though, cause a different reaction. Dairy products—milk, yogurt, ice cream—create dramatic insulin surges without the corresponding effect on blood sugar. You also get this insulin response from some foods that are virtually carbohydrate free, such as beef and fish, which have hardly any effect on blood sugar. When blood sugar remains relatively constant, it allows insulin to use the nutrients in your blood to build and repair cells, including muscle tissue.

That's why the Abs Diet centers around high-fiber, nutrient-dense foods that are also the ones thought to be most useful for weight control. Most are moderate to high protein, some are high in dairy calcium, and those that are carb based emphasize fiber and other important nutrients.

With more and more evidence showing that a high-carbohydrate diet helps promote fat storage (unless you run marathons), it's becoming more accepted that low-carbohydrate diets work in helping people control weight. A study in the journal *Metabolism* confirmed that very stance. Researchers at the University of Connecticut found that subjects who ate only 46 grams of carbohydrates a day—about 8 percent of calories—lost 7 pounds of fat and gained 2 pounds of muscle in 6 weeks. But you can make a major mistake by eliminating carbohydrates entirely. Many carbohydrates—like fruits, vegetables, whole grains, and beans—help protect you against cancer and other diseases, and some carbs contain nutrients like fiber, which helps you lose and control weight.

Traditionally, the confusion about carbohydrates has centered around finding ways to classify them and figuring out which ones are better for your body. It used to be that we thought of carbohydrates only by their molecular structure—either simple or complex. Simple indicates a carb with one or two sugar molecules—things like sucrose (table sugar), fructose (in fruit), and lactose (in dairy products). Complex carbohydrates are ones that include more than two sugar molecules—like pasta, rice, bread, and potatoes. The flaw is that you can't generalize and say a carbohydrate is good or bad for you based simply on its molecular structure. For example, an apple contains nutrients and helps keep you lean; sugar does not. Both are simple carbs, but they're hardly comparable in nutritional value.

Instead, the way to decide what carbohydrates are best for you stems from how your body reacts to the carbohydrates chemically. One of the tools that nutritionists use today is the glycemic index (GI). The GI assigns numbers to foods that indicate how quickly a food turns into glucose. High-GI foods—ones that are quickly digested and turned to glucose—are generally less nutritionally sound than low-GI choices.

Another term for glucose is "blood sugar." The presence of sugar in your blood causes your body to produce the hormone insulin. Insulin's job is to move the sugar you're not using for energy out of your bloodstream and store it in your body. Here's where the GI comes into effect: Foods with a high GI (like pasta, bread, white rice, and Snickers bars)

(continued on page 50)

ONE TRULY CORRUPT CARB

PLAY WORD ASSOCIATION with *high-fructose corn syrup*, and if you're like me, you say, "Froot Loops." But when nutritionists play the same game, they spit out another word: *obesity*. HFCS is a man-made sweetener that's cheaper and sweeter than sugar. Food manufacturers love it because it enhances their profits, so they add it into an unbelievable number of foods. Cereal. Ketchup. Soda. Pasta sauce. Cookies. Even some meal replacement bars, which are supposed to be good for you, list HFCS way up high on the ingredients list.

We're talking about a processed sweetener that didn't even exist in the food chain until the 1970s. And HFCS is really, really, really bad for you. That's because it's packed with calories, but your body doesn't recognize these calories. In fact, HFCS shuts off your body's natural appetite control switches, so you can eat and eat and eat far beyond what your body would normally be able to handle. You probably know people who can down a 2-liter bottle of Coke in a single sitting. Well, guess what? Before HFCS was invented, humans couldn't do that. Our natural appetite control switches would kick in, detect the sugar we were consuming, and say *"¡No más!"* But by shutting off the switches that control appetite, HFCS—a true junk food—is making America fat. By the late 1990s, Americans were consuming about 62 pounds per person every year. That's 228 additional calories per person per day.

The problem with HFCS is not the corn syrup; it's the fructose—a sugar that occurs naturally in fruit and honey. Corn syrup is primarily made of glucose, which can be burned as a source of immediate energy; stored in your liver or muscles for later use; or, as a last resort, turned to fat. But unlike glucose, fructose isn't metabolized by your body as an immediate source of energy; it's metabolized into fat. While the small amount of fructose you get naturally through fruit and honey won't make you fat, eating HFCS is sort of like setting up an IV that pumps fat directly to your gut. One of the worst offenders is soft drinks: Soda consumption has doubled from 25 to 50 gallons per person per year in the past few decades. So the amount of HFCS we're getting is unprecedented, and many researchers think there's a direct link between the huge amount of HFCS we're consuming and the huge numbers we're seeing on the scale.

Go back to what you know about carbohydrates. When you eat any carbohydrate—whether it contains glucose or starch—your body releases insulin to regulate your body weight. First, it tries to push the carbs into your muscle cells to be used as energy and facilitates carb storage in the liver for later use. Then it suppresses your appetite, telling your body that you've had enough. Finally, it stimulates production of another protein, leptin, which is manufactured in your fat cells. In essence, leptin helps regulate how much fat you store and helps increase your metabolism to keep your weight in check. Like the nosy neighbor who tries to tell you how to raise your kids, fructose screws up a system that was working perfectly fine without it. Fructose doesn't stimulate insulin and therefore doesn't increase the production of leptin—and that's the most important argument against fructose and HFCS: Without insulin and leptin, your body has no shut-off mechanism. You can drink 4 liters of Coke or down half a gallon of frozen yogurt, and your body thinks you haven't eaten since the last time Bill Gates borrowed money from his dad.

Soft drinks are one of the main sources of HFCS, but researchers tried to determine whether soda itself or HFCS was the problem. The verdict: HFCS. In a study in the *American Journal of Clinical Nutrition*, researchers took two groups of overweight people and had one group drink regular soft drinks while the other group drank diet soda (which contains no HFCS) for 10 weeks. The regular soda group gained weight and increased their body fat, as well as saw an increase in their blood pressure. The diet soda group consumed fewer calories than they normally would, lost weight, reduced body fat, and lowered blood pressure.

Even if you aren't a soda drinker, HFCS can still sneak up on you. Here's where nutritional labels come in handy. If a label says "sugar" or "cane sugar," the product contains sucrose, which is a 50/50 blend of glucose and fructose. That doesn't seem to be much of a problem. If HFCS is listed first or second, look at the chart on the nutrition label to see how much sugar the food contains. If it's just a gram or two, don't sweat it. But if you see a food that has 8 or more grams of sugar and HFCS is prominent on the list of ingredients, do what you do when you get turned down for a date: Move along to something else. The body can deal with a little of anything, but when your HFCS numbers start looking like SAT scores, that's when you're headed for trouble. Consult the substitution chart for low-maintenance fixes.

FOODS HIGH IN HFCS OR FRUCTOSE	REPLACE WITH
Regular soft drinks	Unsweetened sparkling water or diet soda
Commercial candy (like jelly beans)	Chocolate candy (check the label; some chocolate bars have HFCS)
Pancake syrup	Real maple syrup
Frozen yogurt	Ice cream
Fruit-flavored yogurt	Organic yogurt
Highly sweetened cereals	Sugar-free or low-sugar cereals
Pasta sauce	Sugar-free pasta sauce
Energy bars	HFCS-free energy bars

are digested quickly, flooding your bloodstream with sugar. Insulin rushes in and says, "Whoa, what do I do with all of this?" Whatever glucose isn't immediately burned for energy quickly starts getting stored as fat. What's worse is that if you eat a carb with a high GI in combination with fat—bread with butter, for example—none of the fat you eat can be burned for energy either, because your bloodstream is so flooded with sugar. Insulin does such a good job of turning this new blood sugar into fat, in fact, that soon your blood sugar begins to drop, and you know what that means: You're hungry again.

If you eat a meal with a low GI (like a balanced dinner of chicken, high-fiber vegetables, and brown rice), the food is digested more slowly. Your blood sugar rises only incrementally, and that slow digestion means that glucose is available as energy for hours and hours. That means you have hours and hours to burn off the blood sugar. Insulin doesn't need to rush in and turn the sugar into fat; it can use the sugar slowly for other construction projects, like building and repairing muscle. Moreover, because your blood sugar levels stay even, you don't turn ravenously hungry just a few hours after eating. You build more muscle, store less fat, have more energy, and keep your appetite under control.

By the way, if all this talk about blood sugar and insulin reminds you of a certain health problem—diabetes—then you were obviously paying attention in health class. Continuing to flood your bloodstream with high levels of sugar, followed by high levels of insulin, eventually trains your body to become less efficient at processing these blood sugars. That's called insulin resistance, which is another term for diabetes. It is a terrible, terrible disease—and it is also highly preventable. In a Harvard study, those who ate foods with the lowest GIs, like whole-wheat bread, were 37 percent less likely to develop diabetes than those who ate high-GI foods, such as white rice. For more information on battling diabetes, see our Health Bulletin on page 66.

It's hard to generalize about which carbs are high on the GI list and which are low because glycemic index is simply a measure of time—that is, how long it takes 50 grams of the food's carbohydrates to turn into blood sugar, regardless of serving size. It's a measure, for instance, of the carb-to-sugar conversion time for a whole apple or watermelon, but it doesn't tell you how much carb is in one serving of the food. Nobody eats a whole watermelon anyway.

That's why one latest advancement in food science is to look at a meal's glycemic load (GL). The GL considers both the GI of a food and the amount of carbs in one serving of that food. It helps you gauge the glycemic effect, or the projected elevation of blood glucose, that food will cause.

The higher a food's GL, the more it will cause your blood sugar to spike, and the less control you'll have over your energy levels and your appetite. But considering the GL is only one aspect of creating a balanced diet. "It's better to have a high-GL diet than one full of saturated fat," says Jennie Brand-Miller, PhD, professor of human nutrition at the University of Sydney and author of the International Table of Glycemic Index and Glycemic Load. "Aiming for the lowest GL possible is not a good move because that means you'll be eating too little carbohydrate and too much fat—probably saturated fat." Instead, to maintain your body's best glycemic response, center your meals around foods with GLs of 19 or less and shoot for a GL of less than 120 for the whole day.

Sound confusing? It doesn't need to be. The Abs Diet Powerfoods and the Abs Diet recipes all have low to moderate glycemic loads. All you have to do is follow the plan. And on those occasions when you are stuck and need to choose between two or more foods, refer to the chart on page 49.

Calcium: The Future of Fat Fighting

YOU'VE SEEN MORE than enough milk mustaches to know that calcium strengthens your bones, but did you know that calcium can also flatten your belly? Researchers at Harvard Medical School showed that those who ate three servings of dairy a day—which in conjunction with other foods provides about 1,200 milligrams of calcium (about the daily recommendation)—were 60 percent less likely to be overweight. In studies at the University of Tennessee, researchers put women on diets that were 500 calories a day less than what they were used to eating. Yup, the women lost weight—about 1 pound of fat a week. But when researchers

(continued on page 56)

ABS DIET HEALTH BULLETIN

WHAT THE HECK IS . . . HIGH CHOLESTEROL?

Cholesterol is a soft, waxy substance found among the lipids (fats) in the bloodstream and in all your body's cells. For all the bad press it gets, the fact is that you need cholesterol because your body uses it to form cell membranes, create hormones, and perform several other crucial maintenance operations. But a high level of cholesterol in the blood—hypercholesterolemia—is a major risk factor for coronary heart disease, which leads to heart attack.

You get cholesterol in two ways. The body—mainly the liver—produces varying amounts, usually about 1,000 milligrams a day. But when you consume foods high in saturated fats—particularly trans fats—your body goes cholesterol crazy, pumping out more than you could ever use. Some foods also contain cholesterol, especially egg yolks, meat, poultry, fish, seafood, and whole-milk dairy products. But the majority of it, and the stuff I want you to focus on, is made by your own body.

Some of the excess cholesterol in your bloodstream is removed from the body through the liver. But some of it winds up exactly where you don't want it—along the walls of your arteries, where it combines with other substances to form plaque. Plaque is wack for several reasons: First, it raises blood pressure by making your heart work harder to get blood through your suddenly narrower vessels, which can eventually wear out your ticker. Second, plaque can break off its little perch and tumble through your bloodstream, eventually forming a clot that can lead to stroke, paralysis, death, and other annoyances.

Inside your body, a war is raging right now between two factions of specialized sherpas called lipoproteins that are moving cholesterol around your insides according to their own specialized agendas. There are several kinds, but the ones to focus on are the Jekyll and Hyde of health, HDL (high-density or "helpful" lipoprotein) and LDL (low-density or "lazy" lipoprotein) cholesterol.

The good guy: HDL cholesterol. About one-fourth to one-third of blood cholesterol is carried by helpful HDL. HDL wants to help you out by picking up cholesterol and getting it the hell out of your bloodstream by carrying it back to the liver, where it's passed from the body. That's good. Some experts believe that HDL removes excess cholesterol from plaques and thus slows their growth. That's really good. A high HDL level seems to protect against heart attack. The opposite is also true: A low HDL level—less than 40 milligrams per deciliter (mg/dL)—indicates a greater risk. A low HDL cholesterol level may also raise stroke risk.

The bad guy: LDL cholesterol. Lazy LDL has no interest at all in helping you out. LDL just wants to stick cholesterol in the most convenient place it can find, meaning your arteries. LDL doesn't care that too much cholesterol lining your arteries causes a buildup of plaque, a condition known as atherosclerosis. A high level of LDL cholesterol (160 mg/dL and above) reflects an increased risk of heart disease. Lower levels of LDL cholesterol reflect a lower risk of heart disease.

Simply put, HDL is trying to come to your aid, but LDL is just sitting there, laughing at you. So whose side are you on? If you want to give HDL a hand, start stocking up on the Abs Diet Powerfoods and follow the guidelines of the Abs Diet Workout. Here are some more quick ideas on beating the bad guy for good.

Butt out. Tobacco smoking is one of the six major risk factors of heart disease that you can change or treat. Smoking lowers HDL (good) cholesterol levels.

Drink up. In some studies, moderate use of alcohol is linked with higher HDL (good) cholesterol levels. But take it easy there. People who consume moderate amounts of alcohol (an average of one drink per day for women) have a lower risk of heart disease, but increased consumption of alcohol can bring other health dangers, such as alcoholism, high blood pressure, obesity, and cancer.

Johnny B good. A B vitamin called niacin reduces LDL (bad) cholesterol at the same time it raises beneficial HDL. In fact, niacin can be more effective at treating these things than popular cholesterol-busting drugs, which tend to act more generally on total cholesterol and gross LDL. Be careful, though. While the niacin you get from foods and over-the-counter vitamins is fine, superhigh doses of niacin can have serious side effects and should be taken only under a doctor's supervision.

Tea it up. Three recent studies confirm that drinking green tea can help lower your cholesterol level and reduce your risk of developing cancer. In a 12-week trial of 240 people, researchers at Vanderbilt University found that drinking the equivalent of 7 cups of green tea a day can help lower LDL (bad) cholesterol levels by 16 percent. Seven cups a day is a lot of tea, but even 1 or 2 cups a day could have a beneficial impact. Meanwhile, researchers at the University of Rochester in New York recently determined that green tea extract can help prevent the growth of cancer cells, and Medical College of Ohio researchers found that a compound called EGCG in green tea may help slow or stop the progression of bladder cancer.

Go for the grapefruit. If you want to make one simple dietary change for better health, the best thing you can do is eat a single white or ruby grapefruit

(continued)

ABS DIET HEALTH BULLETIN

WHAT THE HECK IS . . . HIGH CHOLESTEROL?
(CONT.)

every day. New research shows that grapefruit can fight heart disease and cancer, trigger your body to lose weight, and even help you get a better night's sleep. A grapefruit a day can lower your total cholesterol and LDL (bad) cholesterol levels by 8 and 11 percent, respectively.

Cram in the cranberry. Researchers at the University of Scranton in Pennsylvania found that people who drank three glasses of cranberry juice daily raised their HDL (good) cholesterol levels by 10 percent, which in turn lowered their risk of heart disease by 40 percent. Plant compounds called polyphenols are believed to be responsible for the effect. (Note: Cranberry juice often comes diluted, so make sure the label says that it contains at least 27 percent cranberry juice.)

Spread some on. Instead of butter or margarine, try Benecol spread. It contains stanol ester, a plant substance that inhibits cholesterol absorption. A study at the Mayo Clinic found that people eating 4½ tablespoons of Benecol daily lowered their LDL (bad) cholesterol by 14 percent in 8 weeks. When they stopped using it, their LDL returned to previous levels. Benecol can also be used for cooking.

Gain with grains and beans. Researchers at St. Michael's Hospital in Toronto had people add several servings of foods like whole grains, nuts, and beans to their diets each day. One month later, the test subjects' LDL (bad) cholesterol levels were nearly 30 percent lower than when the trial began. In another study, this one at Tulane University in New Orleans, researchers found that people who ate four or more servings a week had a 22 percent lower risk of developing heart disease (and 75 percent fewer camping companions) than less-than-once-a-week bean eaters.

Don't let your tank hit empty. A study in the *British Medical Journal* found that people who eat six or more small meals a day have 5 percent lower cholesterol levels than those who eat one or two large meals. That's enough to shrink your risk of heart disease by 10 to 20 percent.

Refrain from fries. In a study published in the *New England Journal of Medicine*, the exercise and nutritional habits of 80,000 women were recorded for 14 years. The researchers found that the most important correlate of heart disease was the women's dietary intake of foods containing trans fatty acids, mutated forms of fat that lower HDL (good) and increase LDL (bad) cholesterol. Some of the worst offenders are french fries.

Sow your oats. In a University of Connecticut study, people with high cholesterol who ate oat bran cookies daily for 8 weeks dropped their levels of LDL cholesterol by more than 20 percent. So eat more oat bran fiber, such as oatmeal. A study in the *American Journal of Clinical Nutrition* reports that two servings of whole-grain cereal (Cheerios count) a day can reduce your risk of dying of heart disease by nearly 20 percent.

Rise and dine. In a study of 3,900 people, Harvard researchers found that people who ate breakfast every day were 44 percent less likely to be overweight and 41 percent less likely to develop insulin resistance, both risk factors for heart disease.

Fortify with folate. A study published in the *British Medical Journal* found that people who consume the recommended amount of folate each day have a 16 percent lower risk of heart disease than those whose diets are lacking in this B vitamin. Good sources of folate include asparagus, broccoli, and fortified cereal.

Order a chef's salad. Leafy greens and egg yolks are both good sources of lutein, a phytochemical that carries heart disease–fighting antioxidants to your cells and tissues.

Be a sponge. Researchers at Loma Linda University in California found that drinking five or more 8-ounce glasses of water a day could help lower your risk of heart disease by up to 60 percent—exactly the same drop you get from stopping smoking, lowering your LDL (bad) cholesterol numbers, exercising, or losing a little weight.

Give yourself bad breath. In addition to lowering cholesterol and helping to fight off infection, eating garlic may help limit damage to your heart after a heart attack or heart surgery. Researchers in India found that animals that were fed garlic regularly had more heart-protecting antioxidants in their blood than animals that weren't.

Crank up the chromium. According to new research from Harvard, people with low levels of chromium in their systems are significantly more likely to develop heart problems. You need between 200 and 400 micrograms of chromium per day—more than you're likely to get from your regular diet. Look for a supplement labeled chromium picolinate; it's the most easily absorbed by the body.

Snack on nuts. Harvard researchers found that people who replaced 127 calories of carbohydrates—that's about 14 Baked Lay's potato chips—with 1 ounce of nuts decreased their risk of heart disease by 30 percent.

put another set of people on the same diet but added dairy to their meals, their fat loss doubled, to 2 pounds a week. Same calorie intake, double the fat loss.

Calcium seems to limit the amount of new fat your body can make, according to the University of Tennessee research team. In another study conducted at the same lab, people who added three servings of yogurt a day to their diets lost 61 percent more body fat and 81 percent more stomach fat over 12 weeks than those who didn't eat yogurt. A study in Hawaii found that teens with the highest calcium intakes were thinner and leaner than those getting less calcium.

Some researchers speculate that dairy calcium helps fight fat because it increases the thermic effect of eating—in other words, you burn more calories digesting calcium-rich foods than you would if you ate something with equal calories but no calcium. That's one reason why calcium supplements, though good for bone building and other bodily functions, don't have the same effect as dairy—fewer calories to digest, so fewer calories to burn. For best effect, shoot for about 1,200 milligrams of calcium per day.

The Abs Diet recommended calcium-rich foods are:

▶ 1 ounce grated Parmesan cheese (314 milligrams)

▶ 1 cup large-curd low-fat cottage cheese (126 milligrams)

▶ 8 ounces low-fat yogurt (415 milligrams)

▶ 8 ounces low-fat milk (264 milligrams)

▶ 1 ounce (1-inch cube) low-fat Swiss cheese (224 milligrams)

▶ 1 ounce (1 slice) low-fat Cheddar cheese (204 milligrams)

▶ 1 ounce low-fat mozzarella cheese (143 milligrams)

▶ 1 scoop (28 g) whey powder protein (110 milligrams)

Chapter 5

A FLAT BELLY IN 6 WEEKS

A Week-by-Week Guide to How Your Body Will Change

IF YOU FLIP THROUGH THIS BOOK, YOU'LL meet some of the people who went on the Abs Diet—and succeeded. Linda Toomey lost 20 pounds while caring for four young kids. Rebecca Carr became an athlete. And Jessica Guff stopped skipping meals—and started wearing skimpier tops.

Everyone's body is different, and everybody who tries this plan will have a different starting point. But based on the scientific research I've outlined, you can lose up to 20 pounds of fat on the 6-week plan and gain up to 2 or 3 pounds of muscle. For the average woman, that's enough of a transformation to have your abs show. One of the bigger challenges, however, is monitoring your progress on the plan. Here's a look at the four major measurements you can use to see just how effectively the Abs Diet will work for you.

Weight. It's the most straightforward. The heavier you are, the more at risk you are for disease and the less fit you are. It's a good measuring stick to gauge how well you're progressing on your diet, but it's incomplete in that it doesn't take into account the amount of muscle you're going to develop over the course of a plan. Muscle weighs about 20 percent more than fat, so even a dramatic fat loss may not translate into a dramatic drop in body weight.

Body mass index (BMI). The BMI is a formula that takes into consideration your height and your weight and gives you an indication of whether you're overweight, obese, or in good shape. To calculate your BMI, multiply your weight in pounds by 703, and divide the number by your height in inches squared. For example, let's say you are 5 feet 4 inches tall (that's 64 inches) and weigh 155 pounds. So first we multiply your weight by 703.

155 × 703 = 108,965

Next, we calculate your height in inches squared, meaning we multiply the number by itself.

64 × 64 = 4,096

Now we divide the first number by the second.

108,965 ÷ 4,096 = 26

That's not terrible. A BMI between 25 and 30 indicates you're overweight. Over 30 signifies obesity.

This measurement, too, has flaws. It doesn't take into account

---

ABS DIET SUCCESS STORY

"OFF CAME THE INCHES"

Name: Brandee Bratton

Age: 31

Height: 5'1"

Starting weight: 113

6 weeks later: 106

For Brandee Bratton, it was the perfect team approach: She would plan the food and meals, and her husband planned the workouts. What started out as a diet actually became more of a hobby, as the two made the program something they could do together. Starting at 113 pounds, Bratton didn't need to lose a lot of weight, but she still wanted something out of the Abs Diet.

"It's one thing to be petite, another to be strong, fit, healthy, and petite," she says.

So Bratton and her husband jumped on the program (he lost 10 pounds in 6 weeks), and Bratton wound up as a top-10 finalist in the initial Abs Diet muscle mass, and it also leaves out another important factor—weight distribution; that is, where most of the fat on your body resides. But BMI can give you a pretty good idea of how serious your weight problem is.

Waist-to-hip ratio. Researchers have begun using waist size and its relationship to hip size as a more definitive way to determine your health risk. This is considered more important than BMI because of that visceral fat I talked about earlier—the fat that pushes your waist out in front of you. Because abdominal fat is the most dangerous fat, a lower waist-to-hip ratio means fewer health risks. To figure out your waist-to-hip ratio, measure your waist at your belly button and your hips at the widest point (around your butt). Divide your waist by your hips. For example, if your hips measure 36 inches and your waist at belly button level measures 30 inches, your waist-to-hip ratio is 0.83.

$$30 \div 36 = 0.83$$

That's not bad, but it's not ideal. Women want a waist-to-hip ratio of lower than 0.80. If you were to lose just 2 inches off your waist—

Challenge—based largely on the way she transformed the shape of her body.

"For the first 2 weeks, I didn't notice much of a change in terms of weight. What started changing was the inches, and then the pounds just came off at the end—mostly in the thighs and hips area," says Bratton, who also dropped from about 18 percent body fat to 12. "And that was when I really got excited."

Bratton, who enjoyed the interval training and healthy eating, says that the Abs Diet is one that anyone can follow because you're always satisfied.

"This diet isn't a fad diet; it follows all the scientific rules in terms of what to eat and how to eat," she says. "I can say that there's no food deprivation you feel through this. By eating six times a day, you feel satisfied. When it's time to eat, your body gets used to eating at that time, and your body lets you know—almost like it's talking to you: 'Hey, it's been 2 hours; give me something to eat.'"

Now Bratton, who feels healthier, stronger, and likes the new toned look of her body, is studying to become a personal trainer.

"Women often look for solutions through pills, milk in a can, and gadgets," she says. "I advise this program for any woman to invest in her body."

something you can do in just 2 weeks with the Abs Diet—you'd find yourself in the fit range.

  28 ÷ 36 = 0.77

Body fat percentage. Though this is the most difficult for the average person to measure because it requires a bit of technology, it's the most useful in terms of gauging how well your diet plan is working. That's because it takes into account not just weight but how much of your weight is fat. Many gyms offer body fat measurements through such methods as body fat scales or calipers that measure the folds of fat at several points on your body. See your local gym for what options they offer. Or try an at-home body fat calculator. I like the Taylor Body Fat Analyzer and Scale 5553 for its price (about $50), convenience, and accuracy. If you want a simple low-tech test (and this isn't as accurate as what the electronic versions will give you), try this simple exercise: Sit in a chair with your knees bent and your feet flat on the floor. Using your thumb and index finger, gently pinch the skin on top of your right thigh. Measure the thickness of the pinched skin with a ruler. If it's ¾ inch or less, you have about 14 percent body fat—quite fit for a woman. If it's 1 inch, you're probably closer to 18 percent fat, which is also very desirable for a woman. If you pinch more than an inch, you could be at increased risk for diabetes and heart disease.

Body fat percentage can be the most significant measurement because it'll really help give you a sense of how well you're sticking to a plan. As you see your body fat percentage decrease, you'll see an increase in the amount of visible muscle. Experts say that in order for your abs to show, your body fat needs to be about 12 percent. That means cutting body fat by a little more than half for the average woman.

Before you start the plan, it's important to record some of these measurements so that you'll know how far you're progressing. Take one baseline measurement, and then remeasure as needed for motivation. I'd recommend measuring every 2 weeks. That'll be enough time to see significant differences to propel you through the next 2 weeks. (Measure body fat percentage only at the beginning and end of the plan, unless you have easy access to a measurement system.) Any sooner than that, and you're focusing too much on numbers rather than process.

MEASUREMENT	START	WEEK 2	WEEK 4	WEEK 6
Weight				
BMI				
Waist-to-hip ratio				
Body fat percentage*				

Make sure to have the same person administer body fat readings using the same method to ensure consistency.

As with any diet plan, it's also important to develop some kind of quantitative goal—your ideal weight, waist size, or percentage of body fat. The chart above will help you figure out where you need to go.

What's Your Perfect Weight?

IF YOU'RE LIKE a lot of the women I know, you hold one pivotal number in your brain. Not the date of your anniversary or the time your child was born or the number of calories in Mom's meat loaf. It's your ideal weight, a magical number that your mind fixates on as the one that you're truly meant to see when you step on the scale. Maybe you came to that number because it was your weight at age 18, or maybe it was your weight just before you got pregnant, or maybe it's the weight you think you would be if you could just drop that last little extra flab. Whatever the inspiration, you keep thinking that if you could only reach that goal, all your body-image woes would be over forever.

Well, as I've just outlined, weight certainly isn't the perfect measurement system. A lot of things play a role in how healthy you are—from your waist size to your amount of muscle mass. And that means that the number of pounds you weigh can be more misleading than a funhouse mirror. That said, you can come pretty close to estimating your true ideal weight—not necessarily the one blinking on your brain's internal scoreboard but one that takes into consideration a number of different physical factors, including your body type and bone structure. While there's no absolute formula for predicting an exact ideal weight for every woman, the following formula will get you pretty darn close.

Step 1: Do the math. To get a baseline target weight, take the number of inches you are over 5 feet tall, multiply that number by 5, and add the total to 100 for a rough initial estimate of what someone of your height should weigh. So if you're 5 feet 4 inches, multiply 4 by 5 and add 100. Your baseline is 120. But you still need to factor in the other elements that contribute to your perfect weight.

YOUR BASELINE WEIGHT: _____

Your frame can run large or small, no matter how tall you are. Researchers now recognize that having a large frame can add up to 10 pounds of healthy, unavoidable weight to your body. Take that baseline figure you just arrived at and adjust accordingly—5 to 10 pounds more for a large frame, 5 to 10 pounds less for a small frame, no adjustment necessary for a medium frame (see the chart below).

HEIGHT	WRIST CIRCUMFERENCE	FRAME SIZE
Under 5'2"	Under 5½"	Small
	Under 6"	Medium
	Under 6¼"	Large
Between 5'2" and 5'5"	5½" to 5¾"	Small
	6" to 6¼"	Medium
	6¼" to 6½"	Large
Over 5'5"	Over 5¾"	Small
	Over 6¼"	Medium
	Over 6½"	Large

YOUR BASELINE WEIGHT ADJUSTED
FOR BONE STRUCTURE: _____

A body fat percentage of between 20 and 31 percent is considered a "normal" range for women (though as discussed on page 60, you have to be under that to have your abs show). If you can't use calibration tools, but you want a more precise gauge than the thigh-pinch method described on page 60, you can get a good estimation of your fat and how much of it you need to lose by using this formula: First, multiply your BMI (as determined using the formula on page 58) by 1.20. For our sample 155-pound woman, that's:

1.20 × 26 = 31.2

Then, multiply your age by 0.23. So the equation for a 26-year-old woman would be:

0.23 × 26 = 5.98

Add those two numbers together.

31.2 + 5.98 = 37.18

Subtract 5.4 from that number to find your body fat percentage.

37.18 - 5.4 = 31.78

YOUR BODY FAT PERCENTAGE: _____ %

Use the following chart to determine how far over the goal you are. At almost 32 percent body fat, our sample woman is carrying 39 percent more fat than the ideal of 21 percent.

BODY FAT PERCENTAGE	PERCENT OVER GOAL
22	4
23	7
24	11
25	14
26	18
27	21
28	25
29	29
30	32

(chart continued)

BODY FAT PERCENTAGE	PERCENT OVER GOAL
31	36
32	39
33	43
34	46
35	50
36	54
37	57
38	61
39	64
40	68
41	71
42	75
43	79
44	82

Translate your body fat percentage into how much sheer fat you're carrying around by multiplying your body fat by your current weight.

155 × 32% = 49.6, MEANING 49.6 POUNDS OF OUR 155-POUND WOMAN COMES FROM FAT

YOUR WEIGHT FROM FAT: _____

Finally, multiply your percentage over goal from the chart by your total body fat. That's how many pounds of fat you should seek to lose.

49 × 39% = 19.11 POUNDS

Researchers at the New York Obesity Research Center at St. Luke's–Roosevelt Hospital found that waist size correlates better than overall body mass to risk factors for heart disease, such as high blood pressure, blood sugar, and cholesterol. To calculate your waist size, wrap the tape measure around the top of your hip bones. Take the measurement at the end of a normal breath. Then place your index finger next to your belly button and, standing up straight, see how many inches of belly fat you can grasp between your index finger and thumb. If your waist is more than 33 inches and you can pinch 2 inches of fat, you need to lose at least 10 pounds from your current weight, no matter how you've scored in other tests. If you can pinch 1 inch, you need to lose at least 5 pounds.

YOUR BELLY FAT: _____

Your "perfect weight" is somewhere between your baseline weight as adjusted for bone structure and the amount of weight you need to lose as determined by your weight from total body fat and the amount of belly fat you pinched.

Step 2: Change your calories. To consume fewer calories than you burn, it helps to know your metabolic rate—the number of calories you burn throughout the day. Most women have a metabolic rate of just under 1 calorie per minute, or about 1,440 calories per day. To determine your individual metabolic rate and daily calorie needs, multiply your weight in pounds by 11 to get your basic calorie needs (how much your body burns just by existing). So for our sample woman, that would be:

155 × 11 = 1,705

Then multiply your basic calorie needs by 1.6 to estimate your resting metabolic rate (rate of calories burned when you factor in your daily activities).

1,705 × 1.6 = 2,728

Next, factor in your exercise by multiplying the number of minutes per week that you run, cycle, or play sports by 8. As for strength training, if you're doing two sets of the Abs Diet Circuit, add 600 to your previous exercise total. If you're doing three sets, add 840. Divide the result by 7. Then add that number to your resting metabolic rate to get your total daily calorie needs. Here's the math for our sample woman if she does no cardio but does do two sets of the Abs Circuit.

600 ÷ 7 = 85.71

2,728 + 85.71 = 2,813

To get your estimated daily calorie budget if you want to lose 2½ pounds per week, subtract 1,250 from your total daily calorie needs.

(continued on page 68)

WHAT THE HECK IS . . . DIABETES?

If someone you love has ever struggled with the scourge of diabetes, you know what a devastating disease it can be. In the year 2000, diabetes was the sixth leading cause of death in the United States. But chances are that this demonic disorder contributes to many more deaths; it's a leading cause of heart disease, kidney disease, and stroke, and its other complications include blindness, amputation, sexual dysfunction, and nerve damage. It's also highly preventable, and the Abs Diet and the Abs Diet Workout are near-perfect prescriptions.

Diabetes works like this: Your digestive system turns brunch into glucose—the form of sugar your body uses for energy—and sends it into the bloodstream. When the glucose hits, your pancreas—a large gland located near your stomach—produces insulin, a hormone, and sends that into the bloodstream as well. Insulin is your body's air traffic controller: It takes command of all your glucose and directs it into your cells, where it can be used for rebuilding muscle, for keeping your heart pumping and your brain thinking, or for doing the macarena (if you're the type to do the macarena, that is).

But over time, bad health habits can take a toll on your flight command center. Overeating, particularly eating high-glycemic index foods, floods your body with massive amounts of glucose time and time again. Like any air traffic controller, insulin can become overwhelmed when it's asked to do too much all at one time, and eventually, it burns out. Insulin loses its ability to tell cells how to properly utilize the glucose in your blood—a condition known as insulin resistance. After several years, the pancreas gets fed up with producing all that ineffective insulin and begins to produce less than you need. This is called type 2, or adult-onset, diabetes. (Given that poor diet is the major risk factor, it's no surprise that 80 percent of people with type 2 diabetes are overweight.) Glucose builds up in the blood, overflows into the urine, and passes out of the body. Thus, the body loses its main source of fuel even though the blood contains large amounts of glucose.

Two bad things happen: First, you start to lose energy, and your body starts to have trouble maintaining itself. You feel fatigue and unusual thirst, and you begin losing weight for no apparent reason; you get sick more often, and injuries are slow to heal because your body is losing its ability to maintain itself. Second, the sugar that is hanging around in your blood begins to damage the tiny blood vessels and nerves throughout your body, particularly in your extremities and vital organs. Blindness, sexual dysfunction, numbness, and heart damage ensue.

But diabetes is a relatively preventable disease. Exercising and eating right are the two best ways to manage it, and—what a coincidence—that's just what this book is intended to teach you to do. So adopt the principles of the Abs Diet and the Abs Diet Workout, and while you're at it, consider these additional steps.

Get mushy. Oatmeal is high in soluble fiber, which may decrease your risk of heart disease, some cancers, diverticulitis, and diabetes. Mix it up: Eat oatmeal with berries and nuts one day, and have eggs and meat another.

Climb. Yale researchers found that people with insulin resistance—a risk factor for diabetes and heart disease—who exercised on a stairclimber for 45 minutes 4 days a week improved their sensitivity to insulin by 43 percent in 6 weeks.

Steal from the teacher. Researchers at the National Public Health Institute in Helsinki, Finland, studied the diets of 60,000 men and women over the course of a year and found that individuals who ate apples the most frequently were 12 percent less likely to die during the course of the study than those who rarely bit into a McIntosh or Granny Smith. In particular, they cut their risk of diabetes by 27 percent.

Eat the right carbs. Get to know the glycemic index, a measure of how quickly the carbohydrates in a particular food are converted to glucose and released into the bloodstream. In a Harvard study, people who ate foods with the lowest indexes, like whole-wheat bread, were 37 percent less likely to develop diabetes than those who ate high–glycemic index foods, such as white rice. (To find out the glycemic index of various foods, go to www. glycemicindex.com.)

Eat more E. In the alphabet soup of vitamins, E is the one that may prevent the big D. When Finnish researchers evaluated the diets of 944 people, they found that the people with the highest vitamin E intake had a 22 percent lower risk of diabetes than those with the lowest intake. Vitamin E may also prevent the free radical damage that plays a role in the complications caused by diabetes.

Start wining. In a study of 23,000 twins, researchers found that individuals who had one or two drinks a day were up to 40 percent less likely to develop diabetes than individuals downing less than one drink daily. Previous research has linked alcohol consumption to increased insulin sensitivity. Just don't overdo the amount you drink. In a separate study, researchers found that binge drinking may increase your risk of colorectal cancer threefold.

2,813 - 1,250 = 1,563

Start off reducing your daily calorie intake much lower than that, and you'll lose more muscle than fat. As you begin to lose weight, though, deduct another 10 calories for every pound you drop.

I don't mean to hit you with more numbers than Paris Hilton's black book. In fact, it might be easiest to simply focus on one number—six—so that the others will fall into place. When you start to see those six abdominal muscles, it'll mean that everything else has decreased—your weight, your BMI, your waist-to-hip ratio, and your body fat percentage. This 6-week plan will get you there. Here's what you can expect from going on the diet.

WEEKS	WHAT TO EXPECT
1–2	A significant weight loss as your body adjusts to a new approach to eating. Some may see losses of up to 12 pounds in the first 2 weeks (especially if you're walking or otherwise active each day), but 5 to 8 pounds will be average.
3–4	By integrating a modest amount of strength training into your routine, you'll start to feel your body change because your metabolism is working hard. You'll notice an additional drop in weight (most likely averaging another 5 to 8 pounds), but you'll also notice significant changes in your shape.
5–6	After 2 weeks of exercise, your body is primed to make a significant push to drop more fat while also gaining muscle mass. You'll notice that your upper body is more toned and that your waist and other fatty parts of your body are smaller. Depending on your starting point, this is where you'll begin to see abs and really notice even greater effects.

What you'll find so remarkable about this program is how simple it is to follow, how often you'll eat—each meal and each snack is an easy, muscle-building, fat-burning treat—and how unlike any other "diet" the Abs Diet is. Very simply, the Abs Diet is a plan that will ask you to:

▶ Eat three meals and three snacks each day, with each of your meals and snacks including several of the wide-ranging Power-foods discussed in Chapter 8.

▶ Keep an eye out for a handful of diet busters that you'll learn to easily spot and cut down on—not eliminate.

▶ Perform a simple 20-minute workout three times a week to turbocharge your fat loss and muscle toning.

The Abs Diet is so simple that we don't break it into phases, and we didn't design a complex "maintenance" program (just a few simple words of wisdom that you'll find on page 357). The weight loss is yours to keep for life, and so is the eating plan. You won't be waiting for your "diet" to end. You'll enjoy this program so much—and be so wowed by the results—that you'll effortlessly follow it for life.

Chapter 6

SHOCKER: HOW LOW-CARB DIETS MAKE YOU FAT

The Truth about the Trend That's Threatening America's Health

THROUGHOUT THIS BOOK, I'VE HIT you with scientific evidence, persuaded you with real-life testimonials, and referenced study after study to show how the Abs Diet works and why it makes sense for everyone who wants to manage their weight and live healthful, active, disease-free lives. But just for a moment, I want to step away from all the hard science and take you on a bit of a fantasy adventure. Come this way—I promise you'll find it revealing.

First, I want you to imagine that you've taken a time machine back to the Middle Ages. You find yourself at the door of an alchemist's laboratory, where magic elixirs and potions fill the shelves and the echoes of mantras and spells fill the air. You've traveled long and hard, through terrifying dark woods and vast, arid deserts to seek out a Holy Grail of sorts: a concoction that legend says will make you lose weight, magically.

The sorcerer appears, and he holds up before you two vials. The first, he says, contains an elixir that will protect you from most of the diseases known to man. Its ingredients hold properties that will change your cholesterol profile and protect you from heart disease; help scour your body for toxins and protect you from the onslaught of cancer and the side effects of aging; energize your body and your brain, making your thinking clearer and helping to immunize you from Alzheimer's; and, over the course of your long life, control your weight and keep obesity and diabetes at bay.

The second vial will do none of that. It will, in all likelihood, raise your cholesterol profile and increase your risk for cancer, stroke, and heart disease, as well as other ailments. But if you take it, it may help you lose weight dramatically—though only for a short period of time. And there's one more drawback: If you choose the second vial, you can never sip from the first.

Which do you choose?

In the past 5 years, about 60 million Americans chose vial number two.

Now, scrape the dust from the label on that vial and guess what it says? Low-Carbohydrate Diet.

The first vial, on the other hand, brims with all sorts of things: fruits and vegetables, whole-grain breads and cereals, beans and nuts—the sorts of thing that nature intended us to eat but diet plans like Atkins do not. And over the long term, if Americans keep choosing vial number two, I think we're going to pay—heavily.

The Origins of a Sweet Tooth

TO UNDERSTAND WHY carbohydrates are important, we have to take another fantasy trip, this time back to the dawn of man. On the savannahs of Africa, the high plains of Europe, the wetlands of Asia, and the woodlands and jungles of the Americas, primitive man learned how to feed himself from nature's banquet table. He learned how to fish and hunt and, later, how to domesticate animals and grow grain. But since man first stood upright, he has also had a craving for sweets.

As with all things, there's a reason why we crave sweets. The sweetest things on earth, back in those days before Cherry Garcia, were fruits: wild berries, pears, citrus fruits, and the like. Not coincidentally, fruits are also packed with nutrients: vitamins to fend off disease; minerals to assist with cell function; and fiber to regulate hunger, control blood pressure, and help ease digestion. Without our sweet tooth, we would have been happy to eat nothing but woolly mammoth and buffalo meat—the original Atkins program. But nature saw to it that we craved the foods that would make us healthy.

Fast-forward to today, when the sweetest things don't look anything like tangerines. Whereas our sweet tooth was once nature's way of protecting us from disease, now it's the food industry's way of tricking us into it. To satisfy our cravings, we turn to cookies and cakes and chocolates instead of apples and pears and blackberries. That's one of the main reasons Americans today are so fat. And it's one of the main reasons why, in the short term, low-carb diets work.

By limiting carbohydrate intake, diets like Atkins create by default weight loss. If you restrict yourself to just one class of foods—low-carb foods, in this instance—you're bound to lose weight. That's because the stuff you're used to munching on, from the doughnut you nosh in the car on the way to work to the Snickers bar you snag from the vending machine before your drive home, is now voided from your diet. You're eating less food, so you're taking in fewer calories, so you lose weight.

The other sneaky advantage of an Atkins diet is that it focuses on foods that are difficult to prepare and consume. It's easy to pop a bagel or a grapefruit into your briefcase or purse; shove some steak and eggs in there instead, and things get a little messy. So low-carb diets restrict calories in two ways: by limiting food options and by limiting the ease with which we can consume food.

But there are two major reasons why, over the long term, low-carb diets won't work: Mother Nature and the almighty dollar.

Low-Carb Dilemma #1: Take That Out of Your Mouth!

SOMEONE WITH A sound understanding of nutrition and a sadistic streak could have a field day torturing low-carb enthusiasts. Here's an evil trick: Take two pieces of soft, fresh, whole-grain bread. Slather one side with 2 tablespoons of all-natural peanut butter. Now take ½ cup of blackberries, mash them lightly with a fork, and (this is where it gets really nasty) spread the mashed berries onto the other piece of bread.

Put the two sides together, and you've created the world's healthiest PB&J sandwich: 5 grams of fiber (about as much as the average American gets in a single day), 25 percent of your daily intake of vitamin C, 13 grams of protein, and (*sacre bleu!*) a verboten 30 grams of carbohydrate. (Oh, by the way, it tastes incredible.)

Float this concoction in front of a low-carb enthusiast, and you might as well be serving broiled rat viscera. (Come to think of it, they'd probably prefer the rat viscera. No carbs.) The sandwich is achingly sweet, soft, and chewy—a delicious comfort food that, at the same time, is a cholesterol-busting nuclear missile. The fiber protects you from heart disease as well as from stroke and colon cancer. The vitamin C boosts your immune system. And the high-quality (meaning high in fiber) carbs give you long-burning energy and food for your brain. Yet phase one of the Atkins diet bans every single ingredient in this simple sandwich.

Every single one.

In fact, the Atkins diet focuses on something called net carbs that Atkins claims are the carbohydrates that actually impact blood sugar. A rough formula for figuring out net carbs is to subtract the number of fiber grams from the total number of carb grams (the reasoning being that fiber doesn't impact blood sugar, spike insulin, or contribute to fat storage). By that calculation, this sandwich has about 33 net carbs. Phase one of the Atkins diet limits you to 20 net carbs per day. Eat this one super-good-for-you food, and you'll have to fast for the next day and a half to keep your Atkins diet in effect.

Maybe it's just me, but I think this whole low-carb plan is simply crackers. (Oh, sorry—not allowed to eat those.)

See, carbs are not our enemies. As I explained earlier, we crave carbs because we need them to protect us against a host of ailments. The low-carb craze works temporarily not because it limits carbs but because it limits food intake. And if I came out with some crazy diet plan that said you could eat only foods that are high in fat or low in protein or bigger than a bread box or start with the letter P, believe me—you'd lose weight. For a little while, at least, until you couldn't look at pudding, parsnips, and poultry ever again.

(continued on page 76)

WHAT THE HECK ARE . . . CANCER CELLS?

Cancer is the one scourge that can strike any of us at any time in life. It can hit in the places we think about and care about on a daily basis—the skin, the lungs, the brain—or in obscure places we don't even understand, like the pancreas, the kidneys, or the lymphatic system.

Simply put, cancer develops when cells in one part of the body begin to grow out of control. When we're children, our cells are constantly dividing, creating the new cells that help us grow. Once we reach adulthood, that cell growth stops, for the most part. Once we reach our genetically programmed height and weight, cells in most parts of the body divide only to replace worn-out or dying cells or to repair injuries.

But cancer cells act like kids—they keep growing, dividing, and multiplying, outliving our normal cells and interfering with the various functions of the body. The most common type of cancer among women is breast cancer. (The most common type of cancer among men is prostate cancer; the prostate is the gland located behind the scrotum that produces most of a man's seminal fluid.) Breast cancer results in about a quarter million new cases every year.

We don't fully understand what causes cancer, but we do know some of the risk factors: Obesity, low-fiber diets, smoking, heavy alcohol use, overexposure to the sun, and exposure to radiation and other toxins are among the biggest dangers. Additionally, there's a strong link between heredity and cancer; if one or more close relatives has suffered a bout of the disease, you're at increased risk for cancer in general and for that specific form in particular.

I'd like to tell you that the Abs Diet is a magic bullet against cancer, but I can't; while dietary changes and exercise can dramatically decrease your risk for heart disease, stroke, and especially diabetes, cancer remains a bit more elusive. Still, by adopting the principles of the Abs Diet, you'll automatically decrease your risk for many forms of cancer because you'll decrease your weight and increase your fiber intake. In the meantime, you can also follow these additional tips to slash your risk even more.

Color your plate. A 14-year study found that those whose diets were highest in fruits and vegetables had a 70 percent lower risk of digestive-tract cancers.

Order the Chilean red. Chilean cabernet sauvignon is 38 percent higher than French wine in flavonols—compounds called antioxidants that help deter cancer.

Try the cheese platter. A large-scale study of 120,000 women found that premenopausal women who consumed a lot of dairy products, especially low-fat and fat-free ones, ran a lower risk of breast cancer.

Squeeze a carrot. One 8-ounce glass of Odwalla Carrot Juice—pure pressed carrot juice—gives you 700 percent of your daily recommendation for beta-carotene (and only 70 calories). Beta-carotene has been linked in several studies to a lower risk of cancer.

Bite the broccoli. It contains a compound called indole-3-carbinol, which has been shown to fight various forms of cancer. Don't like broccoli? Try daikon, an Asian radish that looks like a big white carrot. It's a distant cousin.

Serve the salmon. Or any other fish high in omega-3 fatty acids. Omega-3s can help mollify your cancer risk.

Order drinks with a twist. According to University of Arizona research, lemon zest and orange zest contain d-limonene, an antioxidant that can reduce your risk of skin cancer by up to 30 percent if you consume quantities as small as 1 tablespoon per week.

Go green. In a recent Rutgers University study, mice given green tea had 51 percent fewer incidences of skin cancer than control mice. Green tea is another great source of cancer-fighting antioxidants.

Get a D. Foods high in vitamin D, like low-fat milk, help detoxify cancer-causing chemicals released during the digestion of high-fat foods, according to a study at the University of Texas Southwestern Medical Center.

Be Popeye. Japanese researchers found that neoxanthin, a compound in spinach, was successful at preventing the growth of some cancer cells.

Show yourself the whey. Whey protein is a great source of cysteine, a major building block of the prostate cancer–fighting agent glutathione.

Eat the whole grain. Whole-grain carbohydrates are a great source of fiber. European researchers found that those with the highest daily intakes of fiber also had a 40 percent lower risk of developing colon cancer.

Toss in the tomatoes. Tomatoes are one of the best sources of lycopene, a nutrient that has been shown to inhibit the growth of prostate cancer cells. In fact, researchers say that two to four servings of tomatoes a week can cut a man's prostate cancer risk by 34 percent. Even better news: Lycopene isn't diminished by cooking, so pasta sauce and pizza will strike a blow against the disease as well.

You'd lose weight because, by restricting your food intake, I've restricted your calorie intake. And the fact is, when you take in fewer calories than you burn, you lose weight; when you take in more calories than you burn, you gain weight. That's true regardless of where those calories come from. The Abs Diet works both by cutting the number of calories you take in through a sensible-but-satiating eating plan and by increasing the number of calories you burn away by improving your metabolic function. Fewer calories coming in here, a few more burned off there, and presto—weight loss. No magic, no deprivation, and no pointing fingers at the evils of carbohydrates.

The confusion about carbs comes from the fact that in today's society, we're surrounded by high-carbohydrate foods that have had all their positive attributes stripped from them. The refined flours and sugars and sugar substitutes that you find in everything from cookies to ice cream to mass-produced ketchup and peanut butter give us all the calories and none of the nutritional benefits of their original ancestors: whole grains and fruits. The lack of fiber in, say, a plain bagel causes the calories in the bagel to be digested quickly, flooding the bloodstreams with glucose, triggering spikes in the digestive hormone insulin—which then turns the blood sugar into fat cells and leaves you hungry once again.

But fruits, vegetables, and whole-grain bread products have a very different effect on the body: They're digested slowly, giving us long-burning energy. Insulin levels stay steady while fiber scours our bodies for cholesterol and other harmful substances, and the vitamins and minerals inherent in those foods help protect us from a host of ills.

The longer we try to go without carbs, the more our bodies crave them. Eventually, you have to fall off a carb-restricting diet: Your body is programmed to make you seek out carbs, just the way it's programmed to blink when something hurtles toward your eye. It's one of our natural defense mechanisms, and what Mother Nature wants, she will eventually get.

Then again, what corporate America wants, it too will get. Which presents us with part two of why the low-carb craze is a disaster waiting to happen.

Low-Carb Dilemma #2: Follow the Money

REMEMBER WHAT I said about why the low-carb diet appears to work? Because it cuts out a majority of foods that people love to eat and because it makes eating on the run difficult. Those two factors conspire to restrict calories, and fewer calories mean less weight.

Now, here's an easy question: How do food manufacturers make money? By selling you food. So what happens when 60 million Americans decide they're going to stop buying all the candy bars, loaves of bread, boxes of pasta, and jars of sugary spreads that manufacturers have obligingly loaded with carbohydrates over the past half century?

Food manufacturers are going to have to come up with something else to sell. Something they can tout as low-carb, to appeal to Atkins-oriented dieters, but something that's familiar, easy to find, and even easier to consume. And so begins the next phase in the American obesity epidemic.

In February 2004, the *New York Times* reported on the growing trend toward low-carb marketing among restaurants and grocery stores. Retailers are being counseled by their business advisors to open up "low-carb" aisles; restaurants are vying for the coveted "Atkins approved" label to hang in their windows. And in the past 5 years, an estimated 728 new food products claiming to be low in carbohydrates have hit the shelves. Today, you can snack on low-carb candy, low-carb cake, and low-carb brownies, washing it all down with a couple of bottles of low-carb beer.

To get a sneak preview of where all this is going, let's hop back into that time travel machine. This time, we're not going to the storied Middle Ages or the dawn of humanity . . . we're just going back about 10 years or so, to the beginnings of the last diet craze that swept the nation: the low-fat craze.

It's the early 1990s. The low-carb craze hasn't yet begun to blossom. (For better or worse, neither has Britney Spears.) But another mantra has begun to take hold in American society: Eat less fat.

This directive comes not from a book-peddling diet doc but from the US government, in the form of a revised food pyramid designed by the

Food and Drug Administration. Fat has been fingered as the root of all dietary evils: Simply put, fatty foods translate into fatty people. Diet experts race to defend this idea, which on the face of it seems pretty logical: Dietary fat is more easily transformed into body fat, whereas carbohydrates are preferentially burned off for energy. Hence, swap your fat calories for carb calories, and voilà, you've entered the magical weight-loss zone.

Quickly, food manufacturers move to capitalize on these exciting developments. As sales of fat-free milk rise, packages of reduced-fat, low-fat, and fat-free cheeses, spreads, yogurts, ice creams, cakes, and cookies begin to fill the supermarket shelves. Some taste okay. Some taste like sugar-crusted cardboard. But what the heck—no fat, no foul. *Carbo-loading* becomes a byword of amateur athletes all across the country.

However, this whole low-fat theory comes with one big but. (Actually, it comes with millions of big butts, as the obesity rate has risen 15 percent in the past 10 years.) Like today's low-carb craze, the low-fat craze originally appears to work because it creates a restrictive eating program that eliminates certain foods and, hence, a certain number of calories. If you suddenly have to cut out countless steaks, baked goods, slabs of butter, nuts, dairy products, and desserts, presto—you lose weight.

But, as with carbohydrates, our bodies crave fat. Fatty foods (beef, fish, and dairy products, for instance) are usually high in muscle-building proteins and supply critical vitamins and minerals (the vitamin E in nuts and oils, the calcium in cheese and yogurt). So you can go on a low-fat diet for only so long before you wind up facedown in a pint of Chunky Monkey. That's the way Mother Nature planned it.

What she didn't plan for, however, was the craftiness of food marketers. Knowing that low-fat dieters are secretly pining for the old days when a nice slice of cake and a scoop of ice cream ended every celebratory meal, grocery manufacturers go into the laboratory and come out with hundreds of new low-fat foods. And that leads to what should go down in history as The Great SnackWells Debacle.

Nabisco conceived SnackWell's as the ultimate answer to the low-fat diet craze. SnackWell's, which you can still find on grocery shelves today, are fat-free and low-fat cookies that somehow carry nearly all the flavor of full-fat cookies. The secret is that Nabisco loads up the cookies with extra sugar (except in the sugar-free varieties), so you can indulge your sweet tooth without ever missing the fat. How this development plays out in the mind of the average consumer is simple to predict.

"All I have to do to lose weight is to cut out fat."

"Hey! These cookies have no fat. Let's buy two packages!"

"Honey, did you eat that second package of cookies for breakfast? I wanted it!"

The magic bullet doesn't work, in part because we need to eat fats and in part because we've been fooled into thinking that we can eat whatever we want, in whatever quantity we want, as long as we aren't eating fat. So we scarf down sugar calories by the spoonful, and we all get just a little bit fatter in the process.

Okay, hop out of the time machine—trip's over. It's a decade later and, instead of a low-fat craze, America is caught up in the throes of a low-carb craze. And the same scenario is playing out all over again. Every grocery store and corner deli is filled with products—particularly "meal replacement" bars—that are marketed with bywords like *low-carb* or *carb smart*.

Suddenly, it's not hard to eat low-carb anymore. Today—and increasingly more so tomorrow—we can fill our shopping carts with all the foods we cut out for the past couple of years. Food marketers are altering the makeups of their products, packing them with soy protein and fiber and sugar alcohols—all ingredients that lower the "net carb" impact of the food. Now, I'm all for more protein and fiber. Sugar alcohol, on the other hand, is nothing but empty calories that, in elevated quantities, cause gastric distress and flatulence.

What I am against is the notion that marketers are peddling—that we can eat whatever and whenever we want as long as we're not eating carbs. It is exactly the same trap we fell into 10 years ago: a restrictive diet that offers short-term success, turned into a food craze that guarantees even greater health risks and higher obesity rates.

And that's a time travel destination no one wants to arrive at.

Chapter 7

THE ABS DIET NUTRITION PLAN

The Powerfoods and System That Will Change Your Body

IN THE PREVIOUS CHAPTERS, I GAVE AN overview of some cool science—how your body reacts to different foods, why some fats are good and others are evil, and how some foods such as dairy products have a secret ingredient that helps your body burn fat. Science can be fun, but by this point in the book, you've probably got one burning question in your mind:

Hey, when can we eat?

So let's get right to it, because eating more of the right foods more often is the basis of the Abs Diet. Remember:

MORE FOOD + MORE MUSCLE = LESS FLAB

That's why the Abs Diet isn't a diet you'll feel you "have to" stick to. It's one you'll want to stick to.

Guideline 1: Eat Six Meals a Day

WE'RE SO USED to hearing people talk about eating less food that it's become weight-loss doctrine. But as you remember from the physiology of metabolism, you have to eat more often to change your body composition. The new philosophy I want you to keep in mind is "energy balance."

Researchers at Georgia State University developed a technique to measure hourly energy balance—that is, how many calories you're burning versus how many calories you're taking in. The researchers found that if you keep your hourly surplus or deficit within 300 to 500 calories at all times, you will best be able to change your body composition by losing fat and adding lean muscle mass. Those subjects with the largest energy imbalances (those who were over 500 calories in either ingestion or expenditure) were the fattest, while those with the most balanced energy levels were the leanest. So if you eat only your three squares a day, you're creating terrific imbalances in your energy levels. Between meals, you're burning many more calories than you're taking in. At mealtimes, you're taking in many more than you're burning. Research shows that this kind of eating plan is great—if your dream is to be a high-rise condo. But if you want to look slimmer, feel fitter, and—not coincidentally—live longer, then you need to eat more often. In the same study, subjects who added three snacks a day to three regular meals balanced out their energy better, lost fat, and increased lean body mass (as well as increased their power and endurance).

In a similar study, researchers in Japan found that athletes who ate the same amount of calories a day from either two or six meals both lost an average of 11 pounds in 2 weeks. But the ones who ate six meals a day lost 3 pounds more fat and 3 pounds less muscle than the ones who ate only two meals.

There's science to support the fact that more meals work, but the plain-speak reason it works is because it does something that many diets don't do: It keeps you full and satiated, which will reduce the likelihood of a diet-destroying binge.

How it works: For scheduling purposes, alternate your larger meals with smaller snacks. Eat two of your snacks roughly 2 hours before lunch and dinner, and one snack roughly 2 hours after dinner.

Sample time schedule:

8 a.m.: breakfast

11 a.m.: snack

1 p.m.: lunch

4 p.m.: snack

6 p.m.: dinner

8 p.m.: snack

For examples of weekly meal plans, check out Chapter 10. These plans are not something you need to stick to religiously, just a suggestion for how you can make the Abs Diet work for you. It also shows how to incorporate the recipes you'll find in Chapter 9 into your everyday life.

Guideline 2: Make These 12 Abs Diet Powerfoods the Staples of Your Diet

THE ABS DIET will teach you to focus on (not restrict yourself to) a handful of food types—the Abs Diet Power 12—to fulfill your core nutritional needs. These foods are all good for you. They're so good, in fact, that they'll just about single-handedly exchange your fat for a toned, lean body (provided you've kept your receipt). Just as important, I've designed the Power 12 to include literally thousands of food combinations. There are hundreds of dairy products, fruits and vegetables, lean meats, and other choices to satisfy your tastes. Incorporating these Powerfoods into your six meals a day will satiate your tastes and cravings and keep you from feasting on the dangerous fat promoters in your diet.

You'll read more about these Powerfoods in Chapter 8. For now, I just want you to remember:

Almonds and other nuts

Beans and legumes

Spinach and other green vegetables

Dairy (fat-free or low-fat milk, yogurt, cheese)

Instant oatmeal (unsweetened, unflavored)

Eggs

Turkey and other lean meats

Peanut butter

Olive oil

Whole-grain breads and cereals

Extra-protein (whey) powder

Raspberries and other berries

Guideline 3: Drink Smoothies Regularly

WITH SCHEDULES the way they are today, it's no wonder that your definition of a kitchen appliance is the take-out menu. No matter how busy you
are, you need to squeeze one appliance into your life: the blender. I don't
care how many speeds it has or how it looks, and I couldn't tell you the
difference between a mince and a frappe. All I care about is how much
stuff I can put in it and how good the stuff tastes when it comes out. (One
thing I do recommend: Get a blender with at least 400 watts, which will
give it the power to handle chopping ice and shredding fruit and to out-
last any Jimmy Buffett fans who might drop by unexpectedly.)

When you consider that changing your body takes time, motivation,
and knowledge, consider your blender to be one of your most powerful
tools in this plan. Smoothies made with a mixture of the Abs Diet Powerfoods can act as meal substitutions and as potent snacks, and they
work for a few reasons.

▶ They require little time.

▶ Adding berries, flavored whey powder, or peanut butter will
make them taste like dessert, which will satisfy your sweet
cravings.

▶ Their thickness takes up a lot of space in your stomach.

Here's the evidence showing these blended power drinks will help
you control your weight.

▶ Researchers at Purdue University in West Lafayette, Indiana,
found that people stayed fuller longer when they drank thick

drinks than when they drank thin ones—even when calories, temperatures, and amounts were equal.

▶ A Penn State study found that people who drank yogurt shakes that had been blended until they doubled in volume ate 96 fewer calories a day than those who drank shakes of normal thickness.

▶ In a study presented at the North American Association of the Study of Obesity, researchers found that regularly drinking meal replacements increased the chances of losing weight and keeping it off for longer than a year.

▶ A University of Tennessee study found that people who added three servings of yogurt a day to their diets lost 61 percent more body fat and 81 percent more stomach fat over 12 weeks than those who didn't eat yogurt. Wow! Researchers speculated that the calcium helps the body burn fat and limit the amount of new fat your body can make.

How it works: Drink an 8-ounce smoothie for breakfast, as a meal substitute, or as a snack before or after your workout.

Guideline 4: Stop Counting

BY EATING the 12 Abs Diet Powerfoods and their many relatives, the foods themselves will, in a way, count your calories for you. They'll keep you healthy and feeling full and satisfied. Plus, the most energy-efficient foods are almost like doormen at a nightclub: They're not going to let any of the riffraff in without your approval.

Of course, that doesn't give you license to speed down the road of monstrous portions. Most of us claim that we watch what we eat, but most of us don't have a clue. A US Department of Agriculture study asked people what they ate, then checked it against reality. The truth: People eat twice the grains, fats, and sweets that they estimate. If you eat six well-balanced meals, your body will regulate portions through things like fiber, protein, and the sheer volume of the smoothies. That said, it's always wise—especially in the beginning of the plan, when you're most vulnerable and adjusting to a new way of eating—to focus on portion control by limiting the servings of some foods, especially the ones with fat (like peanut butter) and carbohydrates (like rice or bread). A good rule: Stick to one to two servings per food group and keep the total contents of each meal contained to the diameter of your plate. A height restriction is in effect. If you do like to count calories, go at it. I'll give you some strategies for doing so on page 152.

Guideline 5: Know What to Drink— And What Not To

I DRINK BEER. I drink wine. I like to drink beer and wine, and gin and tonics on a hot summer day, and a lot of other things. There are health benefits to having one or two drinks a day, but there are many ways that alcohol can get you into trouble. Most important, alcohol—just like soda—adds calories that you don't need right now. These calories are empty calories because they don't actually help make you full or decrease the amount of food you'll eat. In fact, alcohol makes you eat more and encourages your body to burn less fat. When Swiss researchers gave eight healthy people enough alcohol to exceed their daily calorie requirements by 25 percent (five beers for someone who eats 3,000 calories a day), they found that booze actually impaired their ability to burn fat by as much as 36 percent. Booze also makes you store fat. Your body sees alcohol as a poison and tries to get rid of it. So your liver stops processing all other calories until it has dealt with the alcohol. Anything else you eat while you're drinking most likely will end up as fat. In some more indirect ways, alcohol can inhibit your body's production of hormones that help burn fat and build muscle.

I hate to tell you to drink water, but drinking about eight glasses a day has a lot of benefits. It helps keep you satiated. (A lot of times what we interpret as hunger is really thirst.) Water flushes the waste products your body makes when it breaks down fat for energy or when it processes protein. You also need water to transport nutrients to your muscles, help digest food, and keep your metabolism clicking.

If you're serious about shedding belly flab, I'd encourage you to stay away from alcohol for the 6-week plan. At the least, limit yourself to two or three alcoholic drinks per week. The best drinks you can have are fat-free, 1 percent, or 2 percent milk; water; and green tea (or, if you must, two glasses of diet soda a day).

Guideline 6: For One Meal a Week, Forget the First Five Guidelines

I WOULD NEVER ADVOCATE cheating on your spouse, your employer, or your taxes. But I want you to cheat on this diet. I want you to take one meal during the week and forget everything about good carbohydrates and good fats. Have half a pizza, Kit Kats, Alfredo sauce, or whatever it is that you miss the most while you're on this plan. Have it, savor it, and then dig back in for another week. I want you to cheat for a couple reasons. One, I want you to control when you cheat. Plan your cheat meal for the week—whether it's Saturday night out, a neighbor's cookout, or whenever. But if you keep it planned, you'll stick to it. The way to control your cravings is to satisfy them every once in a while. If you can make it through 6 days, you reward yourself and know that 6 days of good eating is a regimen you can stick to over the long term. And there's another important reason I want you to cheat: because it'll actually help you change your body. A successful diet plan is about how you eat most of the time, not how you eat all of the time. In fact, a high-calorie day of eating can rev up your metabolism. Researchers at the National Institutes of Health found that people who ate twice as many calories in a day as they normally did increased their metabolism by 9 percent in the 24-hour period that followed. But here's where you have to show control. I think that this diet plan allows you to have plenty of foods that are both good and good for you, but I know you will crave other foods that don't fit into our guidelines. Think of this cheat meal as the carrot at the end of a good week of eating. I encourage you to enjoy your meal of gluttony, and please, don't make the carrot literally a carrot.

SMART SUBSTITUTIONS

INSTEAD OF . . .	HAVE . . .	CALORIES SAVED
Sweet-and-sour pork	Beef with broccoli	480
8 jalapeño poppers	8 mozzarella sticks	345
Stuffed shells	Lasagna	295
Steak sandwich	Hamburger	208
Ham-and-cheese omelet	4 slices of bacon and 2 fried eggs	130
12-oz filet mignon	12-oz New York strip	120
Chocolate cake	Pecan pie	120
Turkey club (with mayo and bacon) with chips	Turkey dinner with mashed potatoes and stuffing	115

Chapter 8

THE ABS DIET POWER 12

Meet the Powerfoods That Will Shrink Your Belly and Keep You Healthy for Life

IN THE PREVIOUS CHAPTER, I GAVE YOU the six guidelines for following the Abs Diet and touched briefly on the Abs Diet Power 12. Now I want you to meet each of these 12 superheroes up close.

These 12 foods make up a large part of your diet. The more of these foods you eat, the better your body will be able to increase lean muscle mass and avoid storing fat. Though you can base entire meals and snacks around these foods, you don't have to. But do follow these guidelines.

▶ Incorporate two or three of these foods into each of your three major meals and at least one of them into each of your three snacks.

▶ Diversify your food at every meal to get a combination of protein, carbohydrates, and fat.

▶ Make sure you sneak a little bit of protein into each snack.

How to read the key: For at-a-glance scanning, I've included the following icons under the descriptions of each of the Abs Diet Power-foods. Each icon demonstrates which important roles each food can help play in maintaining optimum health.

Builds muscle: Foods rich in muscle-building plant and animal proteins qualify for this seal of approval, as do foods rich in certain minerals linked to proper muscle maintenance, such as magnesium.

Helps promote weight loss: Foods high in calcium and fiber (both of which protect against obesity) as well as foods that help build fat-busting muscle tissue earn this badge of respect.

Strengthens bone: Calcium and vitamin D are the most important bone builders, and they protect the body against osteoporosis. But beware: High levels of sodium can leach calcium out of bone tissue. Fortunately, all of the Powerfoods are naturally low in sodium.

Lowers blood pressure: Any food that's not high in sodium can help lower blood pressure—and score this designation—if it has beneficial amounts of potassium, magnesium, or calcium.

OBESITY RISKS

Almost as important as what you eat is when you eat. Researchers at the University of Massachusetts analyzed the eating habits of 500 women and men and found connections between the way people eat and the risk of becoming overweight.

HABIT	CHANGES YOUR RISK OF OBESITY BY
Eating at least one midday snack	–39 percent
Eating dinner as your biggest meal of the day	+6 percent
Waiting more than 3 hours after waking up to eat breakfast	+43 percent
Eating more than a third of your meals in restaurants	+69 percent
Going to bed hungry (3 or more hours after your last meal or snack)	+101 percent
Eating breakfast away from home	+137 percent
Not eating breakfast	+450 percent

Fights cancer: Research has shown that there is a lower risk of some types of cancer among those people who maintain low-fat, high-fiber diets. You can also help foil cancer by eating foods that are high in calcium, beta-carotene, or vitamin C. In addition, all cruciferous (cabbage type) and allium (onion type) vegetables get the cancer protection symbol because research has shown they help prevent certain kinds of cancer.

Improves immune function: Vitamins A, E, B$_6$, and C; folate; and the mineral zinc help to increase the body's immunity to certain types of disease. This icon indicates a Powerfood with high levels of one or more of these nutrients.

Fights heart disease: Artery-clogging cholesterol can lead to trouble if you eat foods that are predominant in saturated and

---

ABS DIET SUCCESS STORY

"I'M SEEING DEFINITION I HAVEN'T SEEN IN YEARS"

Name: Kristen Hutchinson

Age: 39

Height: 5'4"

Starting weight: 134

6 weeks later: 124

When Kristen Hutchinson came across the Abs Diet, she was frustrated—frustrated that her running routine wasn't keeping the weight off, frustrated that she'd gained back some of the weight she'd lost on Weight Watchers, frustrated that she hadn't found the answer.

"The Abs Diet just seemed to make sense, so I gave it a shot," Hutchinson says, "and it was perfect."

By changing her diet with more whole grains, fruits, and vegetables (and fewer bagels) and changing her exercise program to include a quick resistance workout, Hutchinson knocked off the weight she wanted to lose. She also learned some new things about food. "I realized almonds are good for you. That's a treat every single day," she says.

trans fats, while foods that are high in monounsaturated or polyunsaturated fats will actually help protect your heart by keeping your cholesterol levels in check.

#1: Almonds and Other Nuts

Superpowers: build muscle, fight cravings

Secret weapons: protein, monounsaturated fats, vitamin E, fiber, magnesium, folate (peanuts), phosphorus

Fight against: obesity, heart disease, muscle loss, wrinkles, cancer, high blood pressure

---

What Hutchinson immediately noticed was the upper-body tone—especially in her shoulders and arms. It then worked its way down.

"I'm beginning to see definition in my stomach that I haven't seen in years," she says.

Hutchinson especially liked the fact that the workouts are flexible in that she can go to the gym and use equipment if she wants, or she can do the exercises at home with dumbbells if her day becomes too busy. "I also like all the options for ab exercises," she says. "You could just modify it a little bit and not get bored. I like the variety."

Now Hutchinson enjoys the fact that she's in maintenance mode, as she enjoys a cheat day instead of a cheat meal. But one of the biggest rewards, she says, is that the diet reduced her back pain dramatically. She says that since starting the Abs Diet, she has very little, if any, back pain, and it's one of the many benefits she talks about when she speaks of the diet to others. Hutchinson also has a much greater energy level.

"At almost 40 years old, I feel that I have just as much energy as I did 20 years ago," she says. "In fact, because of the Abs Diet, I am now training to compete for a sprint triathlon this fall. The last one I competed in was 12 years ago. I feel that I am in as great shape as I was then because of the success of the Abs Diet.

"It's a very easy diet, and I've recommended it to so many people," Hutchinson says. "I don't even have the book in my hands anymore because I've lent it to a few people so they could get the same benefit from it that I did."

Sidekicks: pumpkin seeds, sunflower seeds, avocados

Imposters: salted or smoked nuts

These days, you hear about good fats and bad fats the way you hear about good cops and bad cops. One's on your side, and one's gonna beat you silly. Oreos fall into the latter category, but nuts are clearly out to help you. They contain the monounsaturated fats that clear your arteries and help you feel full.

All nuts are high in protein and monounsaturated fat. But almonds are like Jack Nicholson in *One Flew over the Cuckoo's Nest*: They're the king of the nuts. A handful of almonds provides half the amount of vitamin E you need in a day and 8 percent of the calcium. They also contain 19 percent of your daily requirement of magnesium—a key component for muscle building. In a Western Washington University study, people taking extra magnesium were able to lift 20 percent more weight and build more muscle than those who weren't. Eat as much as two handfuls of almonds a day. A Toronto University study found that people can eat this amount daily without gaining any extra weight. A Purdue University study showed that people who ate nuts high in monounsaturated fat felt full an hour and a half longer than those who ate fat-free food (rice cakes, in this instance). If you eat 2 ounces of almonds (about 24 of them), it should be enough to suppress your appetite—especially if you wash them down with 8 ounces of water. The fluid helps expand the fiber in the nuts to help you feel fuller. Also, try to keep the nuts' nutrient-rich skins on them.

Here are ways to seamlessly introduce almonds or other nuts into your diet.

▶ Add chopped nuts to plain peanut butter.

▶ Toss a handful on cereal, yogurt, or ice cream.

▶ Put slivers in an omelet.

▶ For a quick popcorn alternative: Spray a handful of almonds with nonstick cooking spray and bake at 400°F for 5 to 10 minutes. Take them out of the oven and sprinkle with a mixture of either brown sugar and cinnamon or ground red pepper and thyme.

One caveat, before you get all nutty: Smoked and salted nuts don't make the cut here because of their high sodium content. High sodium can mean high blood pressure.

#2: Beans and Legumes

Superpowers: build muscle, help burn fat, regulate digestion

Secret weapons: fiber, protein, iron, folate

Fight against: obesity, colon cancer, heart disease, high blood pressure

Sidekicks: lentils, peas, bean dips, hummus, edamame

Imposters: refried beans, which are high in saturated fats, baked beans, which are high in sugar

Most of us can trace our resistance to beans to some unfortunately timed intestinal upheaval (third-grade math class, a first date gone awry). But beans are, as the song says, good for your heart; the more you eat them, the more you'll be able to control your hunger. Black, lima, pinto, garbanzo—you pick the bean (as long as it's not refried—refried beans are loaded with fat). Beans are a low-calorie food packed with protein, fiber, and iron—ingredients crucial for building muscle and losing weight. Gastrointestinal disadvantages notwithstanding, they serve as one of the key members of the Abs Diet cabinet because of all their nutritional power. In fact, you can swap in a bean-heavy dish for a meat-heavy dish a couple of times per week; you'll be lopping a lot of saturated fat out of your diet and replacing it with higher amounts of fiber.

The best beans for your diet are:

▶ Soybeans

▶ Pinto beans

▶ Chickpeas (garbanzo beans)

▶ Navy beans

▶ Black beans

▶ White beans

▶ Kidney beans

▶ Lima beans

#3: Spinach and Other Green Vegetables

Superpowers: neutralize free radicals, which are molecules that accelerate the aging process

Secret weapons: vitamins including A, C, and K; folate; minerals including calcium and magnesium; fiber; beta-carotene

Fight against: cancer, heart disease, stroke, obesity, osteoporosis

Sidekicks: cruciferous vegetables like broccoli and brussels sprouts; green, yellow, red, and orange vegetables like asparagus, peppers, and yellow beans

Imposters: none, as long as you don't fry them or smother them in fatty cheeses

You know vegetables are packed with important nutrients, but they're also a critical part of your body-changing diet. I like spinach in particular because one serving supplies nearly a full day's worth of vitamin A and half of your vitamin C. It's also loaded with folate—a vitamin that protects against heart disease, stroke, and colon cancer. To incorporate it, you can take the fresh stuff and use it as lettuce on a sandwich or try stir-frying it with a little fresh garlic and olive oil.

Another potent power vegetable is broccoli. It's high in fiber and more densely packed with vitamins and minerals than almost any other food. For instance, it contains nearly 90 percent of the vitamin C of fresh orange juice and almost half as much calcium as milk. It is also a powerful defender against diseases like cancer because it increases the enzymes that help detoxify carcinogens. Tip: With broccoli, you can skip

LEAN GREEN MACHINES

Essentially, iceberg lettuce is the nutritional equivalent of a plastic office plant; it adds a little color, but mostly it just takes up space. Iceberg may be cheap and plentiful, but it contains almost no fiber, vitamins, or minerals. If you're going to eat salad, you might as well eat the power salad. Check out this green dream team.

The cancer killer: romaine. This celery-flavored green is one of the best vegetable sources of beta-carotene—712 micrograms per cup. A University of Illinois study showed that high levels of beta-carotene inhibited the growth of prostate cancer cells by 50 percent.

The bone builder: arugula. One cup of these mustard-flavored leaves has 10 percent of the bone-building mineral found in a glass of whole milk and 100 percent less saturated fat. There's also some magnesium in every bite, for more protection against osteoporosis.

The pipe protector: watercress. It's a pepper-flavored HEPA filter for your body. Watercress contains phytochemicals that may prevent cigarette smoke and other airborne pollutants from causing lung cancer.

The heart healer: endive. It's slightly bitter and a little crisp, and it offers twice the fiber of iceberg lettuce. A cup of endive also provides almost 20 percent of your daily requirement of folate. People who don't get enough of this essential B vitamin may have a 50 percent greater risk of developing heart disease.

The brain booster: mustard greens. These spicy, crunchy greens are packed with the amino acid tyrosine. In a recent US military study, researchers found that eating a tyrosine-rich meal an hour before taking a test helped soldiers significantly improve both their memories and their concentration.

The antiaging agent: bok choy. Think of it as a cabbage-flavored multi-vitamin. A bowl of bok choy has 23 percent of your daily requirement of vitamin A and a third of your vitamin C, along with three tongue-twisting, cancer-fighting, age-reducing phytochemicals: flavonoids, isothiocyanates, and dithiolthione.

The sight sharpener: spinach. Spinach is a top source of lutein and zeaxanthin, two powerful antioxidants that protect your vision from the ravages of old age. A Tufts University study found that frequent spinach eaters had a 43 percent lower risk of age-related macular degeneration.

The pressure punisher: kohlrabi. Kohlrabi tastes like the love child from a tryst between a cabbage and a turnip. Each serving contains nearly 25 percent of your daily requirement of potassium (to help keep a lid on your blood pressure), along with glucosinolate, a phytochemical that may prevent some cancers.

the stalks. The florets have three times as much beta-carotene as the stems, and they're also a great source of other antioxidants.

If you hate vegetables, you can learn to hide them but still reap the benefits. Try pureeing them and adding them to marinara sauce or chili. The more you chop and puree vegetables, the more invisible they become and the easier it is for your body to absorb them. With broccoli, sauté it in garlic and olive oil, then douse it with hot sauce.

#4: Dairy (Fat-Free or Low-Fat Milk, Yogurt, Cheese, and Cottage Cheese)

Superpowers: builds strong bones, fires up weight loss

Secret weapons: calcium, vitamins A and B$_{12}$, riboflavin, phosphorus, potassium

Fights against: osteoporosis, obesity, high blood pressure, cancer

Sidekicks: none

Imposters: whole milk, frozen yogurt

Dairy is nutrition's version of a typecast actor. It gets so much attention for one thing it does well—strengthening bones—that it gets little or no attention for all the other stuff it does well. It's about time for dairy to accept a breakout role as a vehicle for weight loss. Just take a look at the mounting evidence: A University of Tennessee study found that dieters who consumed between 1,200 and 1,300 milligrams of calcium a day lost nearly twice as much weight as dieters getting less calcium. In a Purdue University study of 54 people, those who took in 1,000 milligrams of calcium a day (about 3 cups of fat-free milk) gained less weight over 2 years than those with low-calcium diets. Researchers think that calcium probably prevents weight gain by increasing the breakdown of body fat and hampering its formation. Low-fat yogurt, cheeses, and other dairy products can play an important role in your diet. But as your major source of calcium, I recommend milk for one primary reason: volume. Liquids can take up valuable room in your stomach and send the signal to your brain that you're full. Adding in a sprinkle of chocolate protein powder can also help curb sweet cravings while still providing nutritional power.

#5: Instant Oatmeal (Unsweetened, Unflavored)

Superpowers: boosts energy and sex drive, reduces cholesterol, maintains blood sugar levels

Secret weapons: complex carbohydrates and fiber

Fights against: heart disease, diabetes, colon cancer, obesity

Sidekicks: high-fiber cereals like All-Bran and Fiber One

Imposters: cereals with added sugar and high-fructose corn syrup

Oatmeal is like a gold-medal routine on the balance beam—a perfect 10. You can eat it at breakfast to propel you through sluggish mornings, a couple of hours before a workout to feel fully energized by the time you hit the weights, or at night to avoid a late-night binge. I recommend instant oatmeal for its convenience. But I want you to buy the unsweetened, unflavored variety and use other Powerfoods such as milk and berries to enhance the taste. Preflavored oatmeal often comes loaded with sugar calories.

Oatmeal contains soluble fiber, meaning that it attracts fluid and stays in your stomach longer than insoluble fiber (like vegetables). Soluble fiber is thought to reduce blood cholesterol by binding with digestive acids made from cholesterol and sending them out of your body. When this happens, your liver has to pull cholesterol from your blood to make more digestive acids, and your bad cholesterol levels drop.

Trust me: You need more fiber, both soluble and insoluble. Doctors recommend we get between 25 and 35 grams of fiber per day, but most

(continued on page 100)

WHAT THE HECK IS . . . OSTEOPOROSIS?

On the scale of strength, there's a big difference between the ends of the spectrum. There's the sturdy end—steel beams, diamonds, two-by-fours. And there's the fragile end—eggs, china, champagne flutes. Somewhere in between lies everything else. While it may seem that bones fall more toward the strong category, they're also very likely to swing toward the fragile side of the scale. While bones—which are actually living tissue that regenerates itself to form and build new bone cells throughout your life—are extremely strong (they're the second hardest substance in your body after enamel), your bone mass peaks at age 30. After that, your bones gradually get weaker and weaker, making them more porous, more fragile, and more prone to fractures.

Osteoporosis—a type of bone disease that comes from the thinning of bone tissue and loss of bone density—happens primarily to women because of their typically smaller bone mass (meaning it's quicker for women to feel the effects of more fragile bones), as well as hormonal factors. Women can lose up to 20 percent of their bone mass in the 5 to 7 years following menopause.

But the most important thing to know about osteoporosis and bone loss is that you can stop the decline by building new bone tissue and cells throughout your life. Many medications now help people who are most at risk of developing osteoporosis, and doctors advise getting a bone-density test as you reach menopause. (You don't notice any symptoms with osteoporosis, that is, until you break a bone.) But you can also do a number of other things to keep your skeleton strong. The Abs Diet serves as a great osteoporosis-prevention program, especially for its emphasis on both calcium and resistance training—two of the key components of basic bone building.

Drink more white stuff. And we're not talking liquefied icing. There's a reason why milk gets big play in magazine ads and billboards: It's one of the best sources of bone-building calcium. As you age, your body depletes calcium from your bones, leaving your skeleton deprived and more prone to thinning. Calcium—also found in other dairy products and some green, leafy vegetables like spinach—is the main mineral that helps build and maintain your skeletal structure. You need between 1,000 and 1,200 milligrams of calcium a day. You can get there with a couple of glasses of milk, a cup of yogurt, and a few slices of cheese.

Supplement it. If you're not sure you're getting enough dairy, you should consider taking a calcium supplement to make sure you're hitting the 1,200-milligram mark. Recent studies have shown that supplementing with a calcium pill can reduce the incidence of fractures by about 30 to 50 percent in people with low-calcium intakes.

Show some resistance. Studies have repeatedly shown that you need to include resistance training, like the kind found in the Abs Diet Workout, to help prevent bone loss. Penn State researchers even found that exercise is four times as effective as calcium for creating bone mass. In one University of Arizona study, women who did 20 to 25 minutes of resistance training and less than 10 minutes of cardiovascular weight-bearing activity, like jogging or jumping rope, showed significant improvement in bone density. Weight-bearing exercise—like resistance training and running, as opposed to swimming or cycling, which doesn't require you to hold your own or additional weight—is what helps stimulate bones to grow. Even if you walk, it's important to include weight training for your upper body because walking can't help stimulate bone growth in your arms, shoulders, and wrists.

Add a D. As strong as it is, calcium alone can't help your bones. Your body needs vitamin D to help absorb it. Most people get enough because their skin absorbs it through sunlight, and there's plenty of D in the Powerfoods (through the dairy products and fish, specifically). But as you get older, you may need to supplement with pills or D fortified foods. Aim for between 200 and 400 IU daily.

Watch your protein. Here's another reason why excessively high protein diets are as harmful as chewing thumbtacks. Excessive amounts of protein can cause you to excrete calcium, forcing you to have a need for even greater amounts of calcium. As protein is burned for energy, it releases a substance called sulfate. High amounts mean that the sulfate starts increasing the excretion of calcium.

Use dumbbells. Do exercises that force you to balance yourself—that is, use dumbbells instead of weight training and do abdominal work on a Swiss ball instead of the floor. Better balance won't help you build bone and prevent osteoporosis per se, but it will help prevent falls, which are the cause of many osteoporosis-related bone fractures.

of us get half that. Fiber is like a bouncer for your body, kicking out troublemakers and showing them the door. It protects you from heart disease. It protects you from colon cancer by sweeping carcinogens out of the intestines quickly.

A Penn State study also showed that oatmeal sustains your blood sugar levels longer than many other foods, which keeps your insulin levels stable and ensures you won't be ravenous for the few hours that follow. That's good, because spikes in the production of insulin slow your metabolism and send a signal to the body that it's time to start storing fat. Because oatmeal breaks down slowly in the stomach, it causes less of a spike in insulin levels than foods like bagels. Include it in a smoothie or as your breakfast. (A US Navy study showed that simply eating breakfast raised metabolism by 10 percent.)

Another cool fact about oatmeal: Preliminary studies indicate that oatmeal raises the levels of free testosterone in your body, enhancing your body's ability to build muscle and burn fat and boosting your sex drive.

#6: Eggs

Superpowers: build muscle, burn fat

Secret weapons: protein, vitamin B_{12}, vitamin A

Fight against: obesity

Sidekicks: none

Imposters: none

More and more research shows that eating an egg or two a day will not raise your cholesterol levels, as once previously believed. In fact, we've learned that most blood cholesterol is made by the body from dietary fat, not dietary cholesterol. And that's why you should take advantage of eggs and their powerful makeup of protein. The protein found in eggs has the highest "biological value" of protein—a measure of how well it supports your body's protein need—of any food. In other words, the protein in eggs is more effective at building muscle than protein from other sources, even milk and beef. Eggs also contain vitamin B_{12}, which is necessary for fat breakdown.

#7: Turkey and Other Lean Meats (Lean Steak, Chicken, and Fish)

Superpowers: build muscle, improve the immune system

Secret weapons: protein, iron, zinc, creatine (beef), omega-3 fatty acids (fish), vitamins B_6 (chicken and fish) and B_{12}, phosphorus, potassium

Fight against: obesity, various diseases

Sidekicks: shellfish, Canadian bacon

Imposters: sausage, bacon, cured meats, ham, fatty cuts of steak like T-bone and rib eye

A classic muscle-building nutrient, protein is the base of any solid diet plan. You already know that it takes more energy for your body to digest the protein in meat than it does to digest carbohydrates or fat, so the more protein you eat, the more calories you burn. Many studies support the notion that high-protein diets promote weight loss. In one study, researchers in Denmark found that people who substituted protein for 20 percent of their carbs were able to increase their metabolism and increase the number of calories they burned every day by up to 5 percent.

Among meats, turkey is a rare bird. Turkey breast is one of the leanest meats you'll find, and it packs nearly one-third of your daily requirements of niacin and vitamin B_6. Dark meat, if you prefer, has lots of zinc and iron. One caution, though: If you're roasting a whole turkey for a family feast, avoid self-basting birds, which have been injected with fat.

Beef is another classic muscle-building protein. It's the top food source for creatine—the substance your body uses when you lift weights.

Beef does have a downside; it contains saturated fats, but some cuts have more than others. Look for rounds or loins (that's code for extra-lean); sirloins and New York strips are less fatty than prime ribs and T-bones. Wash down that steak with a glass of fat-free milk. Research shows that calcium (that magic bullet again!) may reduce the amount of saturated fat your body absorbs. Choose cuts on the left side of the chart. They contain less fat but still pack high amounts of protein.

LEAN BEEF (55 calories and 2 to 3 grams of fat per 1-ounce serving)	MEDIUM-FAT BEEF (75 calories and 5 grams of fat per 1-ounce serving)
Flank steak	Corned beef
Ground beef (extra-lean or lean)	Ground beef (not marked as lean or extra-lean)
London broil	Prime cut
Roast beef	
Tenderloin	

To cut down on saturated fats even more, concentrate on fish like tuna and salmon, because they contain a healthy dose of omega-3 fatty acids as well as protein. Those fatty acids lower levels of a hormone called leptin in your body. Several recent studies suggest that leptin directly influences your metabolism: The higher your leptin levels, the more readily your body stores calories as fat. Researchers at the University of Wisconsin found that mice with low leptin levels have faster metabolisms and are able to burn fat faster than animals with higher leptin levels. Mayo Clinic researchers studying the diets of two African tribes found that the tribe that ate fish frequently had leptin levels nearly five times lower than the tribe that primarily ate vegetables. A bonus benefit for men: Researchers in Stockholm studied the diets of more than 6,000 men and found that those who ate no fish had three times the risk of prostate cancer than those who ate it regularly. It's the omega-3s that inhibit prostate cancer growth.

Whether you eat fish or not, I want you to consider adding ground flaxseed to your food. As I pointed out earlier, 1 tablespoon contains

FAT CONTENT OF MEAT (4 OZ, RAW, WITHOUT SKIN OR BONE)

	TOTAL (G)	SATURATED (G)
Skinless chicken breast	1.41	0.37
Veal steak	2.45	0.74
Wild rabbit	2.63	0.78
Lean ground beef	4	1.50
Cured ham	4.68	1.56
Wild duck breast	4.82	1.50
Chicken drumstick	5.05	1.34
Lean pork tenderloin	5.06	1.79
Beef sirloin steak	5.15	2
Beefalo	5.44	2.31
Turkey leg	7.62	2.34
Turkey breast	7.96	2.17
Lean beef tenderloin	8.02	3
Lean pork chop	8.19	2.85
Porterhouse steak	8.58	3
Lean ground turkey	9.37	2.55
Veal breast meat	9.73	3.80
Rib-eye steak	18.03	7.30
T-bone steak	19.63	7.69
Ham	21.40	7.42
Pork belly	60.11	21.92
Cured pork	91.29	33.32

only 60 calories, but it packs in omega-3 fatty acids and has nearly 4 grams of fiber. It has a nutty flavor, so you can sprinkle it into a lot of different recipes, add some to your meat or beans, spoon it over cereal, or add a tablespoon to a smoothie.

#8: Peanut Butter (All-Natural, Sugar-Free)

Superpowers: boosts testosterone, builds muscle, burns fat

Secret weapons: protein, monounsaturated fat, vitamin E, niacin, magnesium

Fights against: obesity, muscle loss, wrinkles, cardiovascular disease

Sidekicks: cashew and almond butters

Imposters: mass-produced sugary and trans fatty peanut butters

Yes, PB has its disadvantages: It's high in calories, and it doesn't go over well when you order it in four-star restaurants. But it's packed with those heart-healthy monounsaturated fats that can increase your body's production of testosterone, which can help your muscles grow and your fat melt. In one 18-month experiment, people who integrated peanut butter into their diets maintained weight loss better than those on low-fat plans. A recent study from the University of Illinois showed that diners who had monounsaturated fats before a meal (in this case, it was olive oil) ate 25 percent fewer calories during that meal than those who didn't.

Practically speaking, PB also works because it's a quick and versatile snack, and it tastes good. Since a diet that includes an indulgence like peanut butter doesn't leave you feeling deprived, it's easier to follow and won't make you fall prey to other cravings. Use it on an apple, on the go, or to add flavor to potentially bland smoothies. Two caveats: You can't gorge on it because of its fat content; limit yourself to just a couple tablespoons per day. And you should look for all-natural peanut butter, not the mass-produced brands that have added sugar.

#9: Olive Oil

Superpowers: lowers cholesterol, boosts the immune system

Secret weapons: monounsaturated fat, vitamin E

Fights against: obesity, cancer, heart disease, high blood pressure

Sidekicks: canola oil, peanut oil, sesame oil

Imposters: vegetable and hydrogenated vegetable oils, trans fatty acids, margarine

Olive oil and its brethren will help you eat less by controlling your food cravings; they'll also help you burn fat and keep your cholesterol in check. Do you need any more reason to pass the bottle?

#10: Whole-Grain Breads and Cereals

Superpower: prevent your body from storing fat

Secret weapons: fiber, protein, thiamin, riboflavin, niacin, pyridoxine, vitamin E, magnesium, zinc, potassium, iron, calcium

Fight against: obesity, cancer, high blood pressure, heart disease

Sidekicks: brown rice, whole-wheat pretzels, whole-wheat pastas

Imposters: processed bakery products like white bread, bagels, and doughnuts; breads labeled wheat instead of whole wheat

There's only so long a person can survive on an all-protein diet or an all-salad diet or an all-anything diet. You will crave carbohydrates because your body needs carbohydrates. The key is to eat the ones that have been the least processed—carbs that still have all their heart-healthy, belly-busting fiber intact.

Whole-grain carbohydrates can play an important role in a healthy lifestyle. In an 11-year study of 16,000 middle-aged people, researchers at the University of Minnesota found that consuming three daily servings of whole grains can reduce a person's mortality risk over the course of a decade by 23 percent. (Tell that to your sister who's eating low-carb.) Whole-grain bread keeps insulin levels low, which keeps you from storing fat. In this diet, it's especially versatile because it'll supplement any kind of meal with little prep time. Toast for breakfast, sandwiches for lunch, with a dab of peanut butter for a snack. Don't believe the hype. Carbs—the right kind of carbs—are good for you.

Warning: Food manufacturers are very sneaky. Sometimes, after refining away all the vitamins, fiber, and minerals from wheat, they'll add molasses to the bread, turning it brown, and put it on the grocery shelf with a label that says wheat bread. It's a trick! Truly nutritious breads and other products will say "100 percent whole wheat" or "whole grain." Don't be fooled.

#11: Extra-Protein (Whey) Powder

Superpowers: builds muscle, burns fat

Secret weapons: protein, cysteine, glutathione

Fights against: obesity

Sidekick: ricotta cheese

Imposter: soy protein

Protein powder? What the heck is that? It's the only Abs Diet Powerfood that you may not be able to find at the supermarket, but it's the one that's worth the trip to a health food store. I'm talking about powdered whey protein, a type of animal protein that packs a muscle-building wallop. If you add whey powder to your meal—in a smoothie, for instance—you may very well have created the most powerful fat-burning meal possible. Whey protein is a high-quality protein that contains essential amino acids that build muscle and burn fat. But it's especially effective because it has the highest amount of protein for the fewest number of calories, making it fat's kryptonite. Smoothies with some whey powder can be most effective before a workout. A 2001 study at the University of Texas found that people who drank a shake containing amino acids and carbohydrates before working out increased their protein synthesis (their ability to build muscle) more than those who drank the same shake after exercising. Because exercise increases bloodflow to tissues, the theory goes that having whey protein in your system when you work out may lead to a greater uptake of amino acids—the building blocks of muscle—in your muscle.

By the way, the one great source of whey protein in your supermarket is ricotta cheese. Unlike other cheeses, which are made from milk curd, ricotta is made from whey—a good reason to visit your local Italian eatery.

#12: Raspberries and Other Berries

Superpowers: protect your heart; enhance eyesight; improve balance, coordination, and short-term memory; prevent cravings

Secret weapons: antioxidants, fiber, vitamin C, tannins (cranberries)

Fight against: heart disease, cancer, obesity

Sidekicks: most other fruits, especially apples and grapefruit

Imposters: jellies, most of which eliminate fiber and add sugar

Depending on your taste, any berry will do (except Crunch Berries). I like raspberries as much for their power as for their taste. They carry powerful levels of antioxidants, all-purpose compounds that help your body fight heart disease and cancer; the berries' flavonoids may also help your eyesight, balance, coordination, and short-term memory. One cup of raspberries packs 6 grams of fiber and more than half of your daily requirement of vitamin C.

Blueberries are also loaded with the soluble fiber that, like oatmeal, keeps you fuller longer. In fact, they're one of the most healthful foods you can eat. Blueberries beat out 39 other fruits and vegetables in the antioxidant power ratings. One study also found that rats that ate blueberries were more coordinated and smarter than rats that didn't.

Strawberries contain another valuable form of fiber called pectin (as do grapefruits, peaches, apples, and oranges). In a study from the *Journal of the American College of Nutrition*, subjects drank plain orange juice or juice spiked with pectin. The people who got the loaded juice felt fuller after drinking it than those who got the juice without the pectin. The difference lasted for an impressive 4 hours.

Chapter 9

ABS DIET DISHES
Using Powerfoods in Quick and Easy Recipes

IF YOU'RE LIKE A LOT OF PEOPLE I WORK with and a lot of people I know, you spend more time in the bathroom, in the car, or on the couch than you do in the kitchen. You simply don't have time to cook. You grab breakfast on your way out; fill up on coffee when you get there; eat lunch with coworkers, clients, or kids; and swing by the vending machine or drive-thru in the afternoon. By the time you get home, the last thing you feel like doing is cooking.

Look, I'm exactly the same way. I don't have the time, energy, or creative impulse to cook. My stove top is more likely to be littered with bills and junk mail than pots and pans, and my oven is more likely to be used for storage than for cooking. (Once, my mom came for a visit and accidentally baked my basketball.) The first time I cooked dinner for a girlfriend, she accurately identified the meal as "some kind of meat."

So what you're going to see on the next few pages takes all that into account—that you don't have the time to prepare lots of meals. If you can operate a blender and a frying pan, you can handle these dishes.

Most of these recipes are ones you can make quickly—some in less than 5 minutes. I also know that you're not going to make every meal, so I've included sample combinations of foods that make properly balanced meals, utilizing the Powerfoods. For the dinners, serving sizes are larger than one, so you can also use the leftovers for lunch. And if you've got a family to cook for, it's easy to double or even triple the recipes.

Abs Diet Smoothies

SMOOTHIES ARE ONE of the best parts about being on the Abs Diet. They take less than 3 minutes to make. They pack in multiple high-nutrient foods. They fill you up. If that's not enough, they can also taste like a five-star dessert. You can come up with your own concoctions by using 1 percent milk, low-fat vanilla yogurt, whey powder, and ice as the main ingredients. Oatmeal and fruit make nice additions, as does a spoonful of peanut butter. Include all ingredients in a blender and blend until smooth. For extra volume, add more ice. Here are some examples.

Abs Diet Ultimate Power Smoothie (number of Powerfoods: 5)

1	cup 1 percent milk	2	teaspoons peanut butter
2	tablespoons low-fat vanilla yogurt	2	teaspoons chocolate whey powder
¾	cup instant oatmeal, nuked in water	6	ice cubes, crushed

Makes 2 8-ounce servings

Calories per serving: 220; Protein: 12 g; Carbs: 29 g; Total fat: 4 g; Saturated fat: 1.5 g; Sodium: 118 mg; Fiber: 3 g

Strawberry Field Marshall Smoothie (number of Powerfoods: 5)

½	cup low-fat vanilla yogurt	1	cup frozen strawberries
1	cup 1 percent milk	2	teaspoons whey powder
2	teaspoons peanut butter	6	ice cubes, crushed

Makes 2 8-ounce servings

Calories per serving: 186; Protein: 11 g; Carbs: 26 g; Total fat: 5 g; Saturated fat: 2 g; Sodium: 151 mg; Fiber: 3 g

Cereal Number (number of Powerfoods: 4)

½ cup All-Bran Extra Fiber cereal	1 tablespoon honey
1 cup 1 percent milk	2 teaspoons whey powder
½ cup blueberries	6 ice cubes, crushed

Makes 2 8-ounce servings

Calories per serving: 145; Protein: 8 g; Carbs: 32 g; Total fat: 2 g; Saturated fat: 1 g; Sodium: 155 mg; Fiber: 9 g

Banana Split Smoothie (number of Powerfoods: 3)

1 banana	½ cup 1 percent milk
½ cup low-fat vanilla yogurt	2 teaspoons whey powder
⅛ cup frozen orange juice concentrate	6 ice cubes, crushed

Makes 2 8-ounce servings

Calories per serving: 171; Protein: 8 g; Carbs: 33 g; Total fat: 2 g; Saturated fat: 1 g; Sodium: 94 mg; Fiber: 2 g

Halle Berries Smoothie (number of Powerfoods: 4)

¾ cup instant oatmeal, nuked in water or fat-free milk	2 teaspoons whey powder
¾ cup fat-free milk	3 ice cubes, crushed
¾ cup mixed frozen blueberries, strawberries, and raspberries	

Makes 2 8-ounce servings

Calories per serving: 144; Protein: 7 g; Carbs: 27 g; Total fat: 1 g; Saturated fat: 0 g; Sodium: 109 mg; Fiber: 4 g

PB&J Smoothie (number of Powerfoods: 5)

¾	cup low-fat vanilla yogurt	½	cup frozen unsweetened strawberries
¾	cup 1 percent milk	2	teaspoons whey powder
2	teaspoons peanut butter	4	ice cubes, crushed
1	medium banana		

Makes 2 8-ounce servings

Calories per serving: 235; Protein: 11 g; Carbs: 39 g; Total fat: 5 g; Saturated fat: 2 g; Sodium: 154 mg; Fiber: 4 g

Summer Smoothie (number of Powerfoods: 4)

⅔	cup frozen strawberries	¾	cup 1 percent milk
1	banana	2	teaspoons vanilla whey powder
½	cup cubed honeydew melon	3	ice cubes, crushed
4	ounces low-fat vanilla yogurt		

Makes 2 8-ounce servings

Calories per serving: 199; Protein: 9 g; Carbs: 39 g; Total fat: 2 g; Saturated fat: 1 g; Sodium: 117 mg; Fiber: 4 g

Belly-Busting Berry (number of Powerfoods: 6)

1	scoop low-fat vanilla ice cream	1	tablespoon vanilla whey protein powder
¼	cup each frozen blueberries, strawberries, and raspberries	3	ice cubes
½	cup low-fat milk		

Makes 1 8-ounce serving

Calories per serving: 251; Protein: 15 g; Carbs: 38 g; Total fat: 4 g; Saturated fat: 2 g; Sodium: 116 mg; Fiber: 4 g

Show Me the Honey (number of powerfoods: 3)

1   scoop low-fat butter pecan ice cream

½   cup low-fat milk

1   tablespoon vanilla whey protein powder

1   teaspoon ground flaxseed

1   dash cinnamon

1   teaspoon honey

3   ice cubes

Makes 1 8-ounce serving

Calories per serving: 250; Protein: 15 g; Carbs: 38 g; Total fat: 4 g; Saturated fat: 2 g; Sodium: 131 mg; Fiber: 3 g

Extreme Chocolate (number of Powerfoods: 3)

1   scoop low-fat chocolate ice cream

1   tablespoon chocolate syrup

½   cup low-fat chocolate milk

1   tablespoon chocolate whey protein powder

½   banana

3   ice cubes

Makes 1 8-ounce serving

Calories per serving: 355; protein: 17 g; Carbs: 60 g; Total fat: 6 g; Saturated fat: 4 g; Sodium: 158 mg; Fiber: 4 g

Pumpkin You Up! (number of Powerfoods: 3)

1   scoop low-fat butter pecan ice cream

½   cup canned pumpkin

½   cup low-fat milk

1   tablespoon vanilla whey protein powder

1   teaspoon ground flaxseed

3   ice cubes

Makes 1 8-ounce serving

Calories per serving: 265; Protein: 17 g; Carbs: 41 g; Total fat: 5 g; Saturated fat: 2 g; Sodium: 136 mg; Fiber: 7 g

Coco Poof (number of Powerfoods: 4)

1 scoop low-fat chocolate ice cream	1 tablespoon chocolate whey protein powder
½ cup frozen raspberries	½ banana
½ cup low-fat chocolate milk	3 ice cubes

Makes 1 8-ounce serving

Calories per serving: 340; Protein: 17 g; Carbs: 56 g; Total fat: 7 g; Saturated fat: 4 g; Sodium: 145 mg; Fiber: 6 g

Lemon Drips and Drops (number of Powerfoods: 5)

1 scoop low-fat vanilla ice cream	1 tablespoon sliced almonds
½ cup reduced-fat ricotta cheese	½ lemon, juiced and zested
½ cup low-fat milk	3 ice cubes
1 tablespoon vanilla whey protein powder	

Makes 1 8-ounce serving

Calories per serving: 387; Protein: 27 g; Carbs: 37 g; Total fat: 16 g; Saturated fat: 8 g; Sodium: 289 mg; Fiber: 2 g

Abs Diet Breakfasts

BETWEEN GETTING A SHOWER, skimming the paper, and the last-minute gluing you need to do on Bub's science fair project, breakfast is the martyr meal of the day. You usually sacrifice it for anything else that needs your attention. But if you had to rank the six meals in order of importance, the first meal would rank first. Breakfast wakes up your metabolism and tells it to start burning fat, decreasing your risk of obesity. The quickest way to incorporate the Abs Diet into your breakfast is to combine potent foods (the Powerfoods) to make meals, such as:

► 8-ounce smoothie

► 2 tablespoons of peanut butter on whole-grain toast and 2 slices of Canadian bacon

▶ 1¾ cups of Shredded Wheat and Bran with 1 cup of 1 percent milk, 3 links of turkey sausage, and ½ cup of berries

▶ 2 scrambled eggs, 2 slices of whole-grain toast, 1 banana, and 1 cup of 1 percent or fat-free milk

▶ Cereal made with ¾ cup of high-fiber cereal, ¼ cup of Cap'n Crunch, 2 tablespoons of almonds, and ¾ cup of 1 percent or fat-free milk

▶ 1 slice of whole-grain bread with 1 tablespoon of peanut butter, 1 medium orange, ½ cup of All-Bran with ½ cup of 1 percent or fat-free milk and ½ cup of berries

On the weekends or on mornings when you can spare a few more minutes, these breakfasts will also deliver the appropriate nutritional punch.

Eggs Beneficial Sandwich (number of Powerfoods: 5)

1 large whole egg	1 slice Canadian bacon
3 large egg whites	1 tomato, sliced, or 1 green bell pepper, sliced
1 teaspoon ground flaxseed	
2 slices whole-wheat bread, toasted	½ cup orange juice

1. Scramble the whole egg and egg whites in a bowl. Add the ground flaxseed to the mixture.
2. Fry in a nonstick skillet spritzed with vegetable oil spray, and dump onto the toast.
3. Add the bacon and tomatoes, peppers, or other vegetables of your choice.
4. Drink the orange juice.

Makes 1 serving

Calories per serving: 399; Protein: 31 g; Carbs: 46 g; Total fat: 11 g; Saturated fat: 3 g; Sodium: 900 mg; Fiber: 6 g

Breakfast Bacon Burger (number of Powerfoods: 4)

1	Thomas' Honey Wheat English Muffin	1	slice low-fat American cheese
½	teaspoon trans fat–free margarine	1	slice Canadian bacon
1	egg		Vegetables of choice

1. Split the muffin, toast it, and spread it with the margarine.

2. Break the egg in a microwaveable dish, prick the yolk with a toothpick, and cover the dish with plastic wrap.

3. Microwave on high for 30 seconds. Let stand for 30 seconds. Add the cheese, egg, and Canadian bacon to the muffin, then nuke for 20 seconds.

4. Add vegetables to taste.

Makes 1 serving

Calories per serving: 300; Protein: 22 g; Carbs: 28 g; Total fat: 11 g; Saturated fat: 3.5 g; Sodium: 868 mg; Fiber: 3 g

The I-Haven't-Had-My-Coffee-Yet Sandwich (number of Powerfoods: 3)

1½	teaspoons low-fat cream cheese	2	slices turkey or ham
1	whole-wheat pita, halved to make 2 pockets		Lettuce or green vegetable

1. Spread the cream cheese in the pockets of the pita.

2. Stuff with the meat and vegetables.

3. Put in mouth. Chew and swallow.

Makes 1 serving

Calories per serving: 225; Protein: 10 grams; Carbs: 42 g; Total fat: 3 g; Saturated fat: 1 g; Sodium: 430 mg; Fiber: 6 g

Change Your Tuna (number of Powerfoods: 3)

2 eggs

2 tablespoons canned tuna,
   drained

½ green onion, sliced

In a microwave-safe bowl, mix the eggs until well blended. Add the tuna and onion. Nuke for 2½ minutes, or until the eggs are set in the middle.

Makes 1 serving

Calories per serving: 189; Protein: 20 g; Carbs: 2 g; Total fat: 10 g; Saturated fat: 3 g; Sodium: 249 mg; Fiber: 1 g

Mint Condition (number of Powerfoods: 2)

1 cup low-fat plain or vanilla
   yogurt

½ teaspoon mint (fresh chopped
   or dried)

1 cup cubed melon mix

Stir the yogurt and mint together until well blended, then toss with the melon mixture until completely coated.

Makes 1 serving

Calories per serving: 208; Protein: 14 g; Carbs: 30 g; Total fat: 4 g; Saturated fat: 3 g; Sodium: 197 mg; Fiber: 1 g

Mo' Feta, Mo' Betta (number of Powerfoods: 3)

2 eggs

½ tablespoon feta cheese
   crumbles

⅓ cup torn baby spinach leaves

1 sprinkle dried oregano

In a microwave-safe bowl, mix the eggs until well blended. Add the feta, spinach, and oregano. Nuke for 2½ minutes, or until the eggs are set in the middle.

Makes 1 serving

Calories per serving: 163; Protein: 13 g; Carbs: 2 g; Total fat: 11 g; Saturated fat: 4 g; Sodium: 205 mg; Fiber: 0 g

Waffles Rancheros (number of Powerfoods: 2)

1   egg

1   whole wheat toaster waffle

1   tablespoon salsa

Crack the egg in a small bowl, stir well until the yolk and white are well blended, and microwave for 2 minutes, 30 seconds. Prepare the waffle according to package directions. Top with the egg and salsa, cut in half, and stack.

Makes 1 serving

Calories per serving: 183; Protein: 10 g; Carbs: 14 g; Total fat: 9 g; Saturated fat: 3 g; Sodium: 263 mg; Fiber: 1 g

Breakfast with Barbie (number of Powerfoods: 3)

1   packet instant grits

4   frozen shrimp, defrosted and chopped

1   tablespoon low-fat shredded Cheddar cheese

1   dollop barbecue sauce

Prepare the grits according to package directions. Add the shrimp and cheese, stirring well to blend. Top with the barbecue sauce.

Makes 1 serving

Calories per serving: 167; Protein: 9 g; Carbs: 31 g; Total fat: 1 g; Saturated fat: 0 g; Sodium: 731 mg; Fiber: 2 g

Corn to Be Wild (number of Powerfoods: 2)

2   eggs

2   tablespoons frozen corn kernels

1   slice tomato, chopped

1   tablespoon black beans, rinsed

In a microwave-safe bowl, mix the eggs until well blended. Add the corn, tomato, and beans. Nuke for 2$^1/_2$ minutes, or until the eggs are set in the middle.

Makes 1 serving

Calories per serving: 180; Protein: 14 g; Carbs: 7 g; Total fat: 10 g; Saturated fat: 3 g; Sodium: 203 mg; Fiber: 2 g

The 'Bama Bowl (number of Powerfoods: 4)

1 packet instant grits	2 strips beef jerky, finely diced
1 teaspoon ground flaxseed	1 tablespoon low-fat shredded Cheddar cheese

Prepare the grits according to package directions. Add the flaxseed, jerky, and cheese, stirring well to blend.

Makes 1 serving

Calories per serving: 199; Protein 11 g; Carbs: 26 g; Total fat: 6 g; Saturated fat: 2 g; Sodium: 700 mg; Fiber: 3 g

Abs Diet Lunches

IN THE MIDDLE of the day, drive-thrus and pizza places can be more tempting than a hot tub at a ski resort. Be strong! You can still follow the eating plan no matter where you are. Grilled chicken and chili are usually good options. In sit-down situations, you can also order smartly without getting tripped up by the quesadilla special. Some good combinations include a salad with grilled chicken or salmon, vegetables, almonds or other nuts, and a sprinkling of balsamic vinegar and olive oil. You can also order a piece of lean meat—either on whole-grain bread or by itself—with a side of vegetables. Ask for salsa or a small side of olive oil for dipping. If you bring your lunch or eat it at home, these are some other options.

The I-Am-Not-Eating-Salad Salad (number of Powerfoods: 4)

2 ounces grilled chicken

1 cup romaine lettuce

1 tomato, chopped

1 small green bell pepper, chopped

3 tablespoons Italian 94 percent fat-free Italian dressing or 1 teaspoon olive oil

1 medium carrot, chopped

1 tablespoon grated Parmesan cheese

1 tablespoon ground flaxseed

1. Chop the chicken into small pieces.

2. Mix all the ingredients together and store in the fridge. Eat on multigrain bread or by itself.

Makes 1 serving

Calories per serving: 248; Protein: 16 g; Carbs: 33 g; Total fat: 8 g; Saturated fat: 2 g; Sodium: 875 mg; Fiber: 10 g

Guilt-Free BLT (number of Powerfoods: 3)

¾ tablespoon fat-free mayonnaise

1 whole-wheat tortilla

2 slices turkey bacon, cooked

2 ounces roasted turkey breast, diced

2 slices tomato

2 leaves lettuce

1. Smear the mayo on the tortilla.

2. Line the middle of the tortilla with the bacon and top with turkey, tomato, and lettuce.

3. Roll it tightly into a tube.

Makes 1 serving

Calories per serving: 206; Protein: 17 g; Carbs: 26 g; Total fat: 7 g; Saturated fat: 2 g; Sodium: 1,270 mg; Fiber: 3 g

Guac and Roll (number of Powerfoods: 4)

1	can (6 ounces) light oil-packed tuna	1	tablespoon light mayonnaise
⅔	cup guacamole	1	teaspoon ground flaxseed
¼	cup chopped tomatoes	2	6" whole-wheat hoagie rolls
1	teaspoon lemon juice		

1. Combine the first six ingredients in a bowl and blend thoroughly with a fork.

2. Split the rolls in half and fill each half with ¼ cup of the mixture.

Makes 2 servings

Calories per serving: 606; Protein: 36 g; Carbs: 58 g; Total fat: 28 g; Saturated fat: 5 g; Sodium: 942 mg; Fiber: 13 g

Hot Tuna (number of Powerfoods: 4)

½	cup chopped celery	1	can (6 ounces) water-packed tuna, drained and flaked
1	onion, chopped		
½	cup shredded, reduced-fat mozzarella cheese	¼	cup reduced-fat mayonnaise
		1	tablespoon lemon juice
½	cup reduced-fat cottage cheese	3	whole-wheat English muffins, split in half

1. Preheat your oven to 350°F. In a large nonstick skillet over low heat, cook the celery and onion until softened. Add the cheeses, tuna, mayo, and lemon juice to the skillet and cook the mixture just long enough to warm it up.

2. Spread one-sixth of the mixture on each English muffin half. Put the muffin halves on a baking sheet and bake for 10 minutes.

Makes 2 servings

Calories per serving: 628; Protein: 50 g; Carbs: 54 g; Total fat: 24 g; Saturated fat: 6 g; Sodium: 1,300 mg; Fiber: 8 g

Yo Soup for You (number of Powerfoods: 3)

½	pound chicken breasts	½	cup minced carrots
1	cup chopped onion	1	cup corn
1	teaspoon olive oil	½	cup canned peeled tomatoes
2	cloves garlic, minced	2	tablespoons chopped basil or parsley
6	cups low-sodium chicken stock		
1	cup canned navy beans, drained	¼	teaspoon ground black pepper

1. In a large saucepan over low heat, cook the chicken and onion in the oil for about 10 minutes, or until the onion is golden brown. Add the garlic and cook for 1 minute.

2. Add the stock, beans, and carrots. Bring to a boil. Add the corn and tomatoes (with juice). Cook for 15 minutes.

3. Add the basil or parsley and pepper.

Makes 4 servings

Calories per serving: 260; Protein: 27 g; Carbs: 30 g; Total fat: 5 g; Saturated fat: 1 g; Sodium: 602 mg; Fiber: 6 g

Crunch Time (number of Powerfoods: 5)

3	cups mixed greens	1½	tablespoons Craisins (dried, sweetened cranberries)
2	slices smoked deli turkey, chopped	1	tablespoon blue cheese crumbles
½	small Granny Smith apple, chopped		For dressing: 1½ teaspoons olive oil; 1 tablespoon balsamic vinegar
2	tablespoons grated carrot		
1	tablespoon diced pecans		

In a bowl, mix together all of the ingredients. Store in the fridge until you are ready to eat.

Makes 1 serving

Calories per serving: 296; Protein: 15 g; Carbs: 31 g; Total fat: 15 g; Saturated fat: 3 g; Sodium: 590 mg; Fiber: 7 g

Hurry Curry (number of Powerfoods: 3)

½ cup fat-free plain yogurt

½ cup fat-free mayonnaise

3 tablespoons finely chopped onion

1 teaspoon ginger

1 teaspoon curry powder

1 pound boneless, skinless chicken breasts, cut into ½" strips

1 teaspoon paprika

½ teaspoon ground black pepper

2 cups cooked brown rice

1. In a small bowl, mix the yogurt, mayonnaise, onion, ginger, and curry powder.

2. Place the chicken in a medium bowl. Sprinkle with the paprika and pepper. Toss until coated.

3. In a nonstick skillet over medium heat, cook the chicken for 4 to 5 minutes. Stir in the yogurt mixture. Cook, stirring, for 2 minutes. Serve over the rice.

Makes 2 servings

Calories per serving: 598; Protein: 61 g; Carbs: 69 g; Total fat: 7 g; Saturated fat: 1 g; Sodium: 704 mg; Fiber: 6 g

The Two Chicks (number of Powerfoods: 4)

3 cups mixed greens

⅓ cup garbanzo beans (chickpeas), rinsed and drained

½ cup diced precooked chicken

¼ cup diced ready-made roasted red peppers

1 teaspoon ground flaxseed

For dressing: 1½ tablespoons low-fat ranch dressing, such as Hidden Valley

In a bowl, mix together all of the ingredients. Store in the fridge until you are ready to eat.

Makes 1 serving

Calories per serving: 391; Protein: 41 g; Carbs: 27 g; Total fat: 12 g; Saturated fat: 2 g; Sodium: 884 mg; Fiber: 8 g

Roll of a Lifetime (number of Powerfoods: 4)

¾ cup diced precooked chicken

2 tablespoons diced onion

2 tablespoons feta cheese crumbles

1 handful romaine lettuce, chopped

1 large whole wheat tortilla

Salsa for dipping

1. Arrange the chicken, onion, cheese, and lettuce down the center of the tortilla.

2. Roll tightly, then cut in half.

3. Place the rolls seam side down on a nonstick skillet heated to medium heat. Grill for 2 to 3 minutes per side. Serve with the salsa.

Makes 1 serving

Calories per serving: 397; Protein: 56 g; Carbs: 25 g; Total fat: 10 g; Saturated fat: 4 g; Sodium: 493 mg; Fiber: 3 g

Popeye and Olive Oil (number of Powerfoods: 4)

1½ cups chopped baby spinach leaves

1½ cups chopped romaine lettuce

3 slices prosciutto, chopped

⅓ cup mandarin orange slices

⅓ cup sliced strawberries

2 tablespoons diced red onion

For dressing: 1½ teaspoons olive oil; 1 tablespoon red wine vinegar; ½ clove garlic, crushed; ⅛ teaspoon black pepper

In a bowl, mix together all of the ingredients. Store in the fridge until you are ready to eat.

Makes 1 serving

Calories per serving: 238; Protein: 9 g; Carbs: 23 g; Total fat: 14 g; Saturated fat: 4 g; Sodium: 450 mg; Fiber: 6 g

Reuben Reduced (number of Powerfoods: 5)

¼ cup canned sauerkraut, drained

1 tablespoon feta cheese crumbles

1 tablespoon low-fat Thousand Island dressing

2 slices rye bread

2 slices reduced-sodium smoked deli turkey, such as Healthy Choice

1 slice low-fat Swiss cheese

1. Coat the bottom of a nonstick skillet with cooking spray and heat over medium heat.

2. In a small bowl, stir together the kraut, feta, and dressing. Spread on one slice of the bread. Top with the turkey, Swiss, and remaining slice of bread.

3. Grill for 2 to 3 minutes per side.

Makes 1 serving

Calories per serving: 335; Protein: 23 g; Carbs: 42 g; Total fat: 9 g; Saturated fat: 3 g; Sodium: 1,625 mg; Fiber: 5 g

The Melon Banquet (number of Powerfoods: 4)

3 cups mixed greens

⅓ cup cubed watermelon

½ cup cubed cantaloupe

2 tablespoons grated carrot

1 ounce smoked salmon, chopped

1 tablespoon pine nuts

1 teaspoon chopped mint

For dressing: 1½ teaspoons olive oil; 2 teaspoons balsamic vinegar; 1 teaspoon lemon juice

In a bowl, mix together all of the ingredients. Store in the fridge until you are ready to eat.

Makes 1 serving

Calories per serving: 274; Protein: 11 g; Carbs: 20 g; Total fat: 19 g; Saturated fat: 2 g; Sodium: 635 mg; Fiber: 5 g

Pimp My Shrimp (number of Powerfoods: 4)

- 3 cups chopped romaine lettuce
- 5 large frozen shrimp, defrosted (with tails removed)
- ½ avocado, diced
- ⅓ cup frozen corn kernels, defrosted

- 1 cup grape tomatoes
- 2 tablespoons crushed tortilla chips
- 1 teaspoon chopped cilantro

For dressing: 1½ tablespoons low-fat ranch dressing, such as Hidden Valley

In a bowl, mix together all of the ingredients. Store in the fridge until you are ready to eat.

Makes 1 serving

Calories per serving: 395; Protein: 13 g; Carbs: 38 g; Total fat: 24 g; Saturated fat: 4 g; Sodium: 439 mg; Fiber: 14 g

Abs Diet Dinners

DINNER IS THE PLACE where most of us wind down and pork up. That's because we spend the day serving others. By dinnertime, we're hungry to have some of our own demands met. On this plan, you'll have already fueled up four times before dinner, so you'll feel pleasantly hungry, not ravenous. These meals give you the taste of sin—without the actual guilt.

Italian Chowin' (number of Powerfoods: 4)

- 1 pound extra-lean ground beef
- ½ cup crushed saltine crackers
- 1 large onion, diced
- 1 clove garlic, minced
- 1 tablespoon ground flaxseed or whey powder

- 1 jar (16 ounces) tomato sauce
- 4 whole-wheat hoagie rolls
- ½ cup reduced-fat mozzarella cheese, shredded

1. Mix the beef, crackers, onion, garlic, and flaxseed or whey powder into golf ball–size meatballs.

2. In a nonstick skillet over medium heat, cook the meatballs until browned all the way around. Drain the fat from the skillet and add the tomato sauce.

3. While the mixture is warming, use a fork to scoop out some of the bread in the rolls to form shallow trenches. Spoon the meatballs and sauce into each trench, sprinkle with the cheese, and top with the top half of the roll.

Makes 4 servings

Calories per serving: 569; Protein: 38 g; Carbs: 65 g; Total fat: 19 g; Saturated fat: 6 g; Sodium: 1,341 mg; Fiber: 10 g

Brazilian Chicken (number of Powerfoods: 2)

1	lemon	1	teaspoon dried Italian seasoning
1	lime		
1	tablespoon ground flaxseed	1	teaspoon hot pepper salsa
1	can (8 ounces) tomato sauce	4	boneless, skinless chicken breast halves
1	can (6 ounces) frozen orange juice concentrate	¾	cup chunky salsa
1½	cloves garlic, minced		

1. Grate the zest of the lemon and lime into a resealable bag. Squeeze the juice from both fruits into the bag and throw out the pulp and the seeds.

2. Mix in everything else except the chicken and chunky salsa.

3. Drop in the chicken, reseal the bag, and refrigerate for a few hours.

4. Grill the chicken, turning and basting with marinade a few times, for 10 to 15 minutes, or until the center is no longer pink. Serve with the salsa.

Makes 4 servings

Calories per serving: 205; Protein: 29 g; Carbs: 18 g; Total fat: 2 g; Saturated fat: 0.5 g; Sodium: 726 mg; Fiber: 3 g

Chile-Peppered Steak (number of Powerfoods: 4)

1 tablespoon olive oil

2 carrots, sliced

1 cup chopped broccoli

2 jalapeño peppers, sliced

2 cayenne peppers, sliced

12 ounces lean sirloin steak, sliced thin

¼ cup Hunan stir-fry sauce

4 cups cooked brown rice

1. Heat the oil in a nonstick skillet over high heat. Toss in the carrots and broccoli and cook until tender.

2. Add the peppers and beef and continue cooking until the meat is done.

3. Add the sauce and serve over the rice.

Makes 4 servings

Calories per serving: 485; Protein: 32 g; Carbs: 57 g; Total fat: 14 g; Saturated fat: 3.5 g; Sodium: 224 mg; Fiber: 6 g

Easy Cheesy (number of Powerfoods: 3)

1 medium onion, sliced

1 small red bell pepper, sliced

1 small green bell pepper, sliced

⅔ cup medium or hot salsa

4 multigrain hoagie rolls

¾ pound roast beef, thinly sliced

½ cup grated reduced-fat Cheddar cheese

1. In a nonstick skillet over medium heat, cook the onion and peppers until tender. Add the salsa and heat until warm.

2. Construct the sandwiches with the buns, roast beef, onions, peppers, and cheese, then warm them in the microwave for 1 to 2 minutes on high, until the cheese starts to melt.

Makes 4 sandwiches

Calories per sandwich: 558; Protein: 35 g; Carbs: 40 g; Total fat: 28 g; Saturated fat: 12.5 g; Sodium: 653 mg; Fiber: 4 g

Chili Con Turkey (number of Powerfoods: 4)

1   pound ground turkey

1   can (14 ounces) Mexican-style diced tomatoes

1   can (15 ounces) black beans, rinsed and drained

1   can (14 ounces) whole-kernel sweet corn, drained

1   package (1½ ounces) dried chili mix

1   tablespoon ground flaxseed

¼   cup water

1   cup cooked brown rice

1. In a large nonstick skillet over medium-high heat, brown the turkey.

2. Add everything else but the rice and cook over low heat for 10 minutes. Serve over the rice.

Makes 4 servings

Calories per serving: 407; Protein: 30 g; Carbs: 52 g; Total fat: 11 g; Saturated fat: 3 g; Sodium: 1,578 mg; Fiber: 9 g

Chicken à la King Kong (number of Powerfoods: 3)

2   tablespoons olive oil

½   onion, finely chopped

1   teaspoon flour

2   tablespoons water

1   pound chicken breast tenders

4   teaspoons chili powder

1   cup spaghetti sauce

9   ounces cooked whole-wheat spaghetti

1. Heat the oil in a nonstick skillet over medium high heat. Add the onion and cook for 1 minute, until browned. In a small bowl, mix the flour and water.

2. Add the chicken, chili powder, sauce, and flour mixture to the skillet. Stir. Simmer uncovered for 10 minutes. Serve over the spaghetti.

Makes 4 servings

Calories per serving: 320; Protein: 31 g; Carbs: 26 g; Total fat: 10 g; Saturated fat: 2 g; Sodium: 360 mg; Fiber: 5 g

Salmon Rushdie (number of Powerfoods: 5)

2	tablespoons olive oil	1	clove garlic
1	tablespoon lemon juice	4	salmon fillets (6 ounces each)
¼	teaspoon salt		Green vegetable of choice
¼	teaspoon ground black pepper	1	cup cooked brown rice
1	tablespoon ground flaxseed		

1. In a baking dish, combine the oil, lemon juice, salt, pepper, flaxseed, and garlic. Add the fish, coat well, cover, and refrigerate for 15 minutes.

2. Preheat your oven to 450°F. Line a baking sheet with foil and coat it with cooking spray. Remove the fish from the marinade and place the fish skin side down on the baking sheet.

3. Bake for 9 to 12 minutes. Serve with a green vegetable and the rice.

Makes 4 servings

Calories per serving: 411; Protein: 40 g; Carbs: 15 g; Total fat: 20 g; Saturated fat: 3 g; Sodium: 231 mg; Fiber: 1 g

BBQ King (number of Powerfoods: 5)

5	ounces smoked turkey kielbasa, diced	1	can (14½ ounces) pureed tomatoes
1	small onion, chopped		Salt and pepper
1	can (3 ounces) sliced mushrooms	¼	cup seasoned bread crumbs
1	clove garlic, minced	¾	tablespoon ground flaxseed
1	can (16 ounces) baked beans	¾	tablespoon olive oil
1	can (8 ounces) navy beans, drained		

1. Preheat your oven to 350°F. Put the kielbasa in a 2-quart baking dish and bake until browned (about 5 minutes). Drain the fat and set the dish aside.

2. In a nonstick skillet over medium-high heat, cook the onion, mushrooms, and garlic for 5 to 7 minutes. Transfer to the baking dish, then add the beans and tomatoes, plus salt and pepper to taste.

3. Bake for 20 minutes or until the edges bubble.

4. In a small bowl, mix the bread crumbs and flaxseed with the oil. Sprinkle over the sausage mixture and broil 4 to 5 inches from the heat, or until the top is golden (about 3 minutes).

Makes 4 servings

Calories per serving: 348; Protein: 20 g; Carbs: 53 g; Total fat: 8.5 g; Saturated fat: 2 g; Sodium: 1,463 mg; Fiber: 13 g

Spaghettaboudit! (number of Powerfoods: 3)

¾ pound extra-lean ground beef

1½ onions, chopped

1 green bell pepper, chopped

2 cloves garlic, minced

1 cup sliced mushrooms

2 cans (16 ounces) whole tomatoes

1 jar (20 ounces) spaghetti sauce

2 tablespoons Italian seasoning

1 package (1 pound) whole-wheat spaghetti

1. In a large saucepan over medium-high heat, cook the meat until browned. Drain the fat from the meat.

2. Add the onions, pepper, and garlic, and cook until tender. Pour in the mushrooms, tomatoes (with juice), sauce, and seasoning, and stir everything together. Simmer. In a separate pot, cook the spaghetti according to the package directions.

3. Serve ½ cup of the sauce over 1 cup of the spaghetti.

Makes 4 servings

Calories per serving: 400; Protein: 28; Carbs: 50 g; Total fat: 12 g; Saturated fat: 4 g; Sodium: 798 mg; Fiber: 10 g

Tortilla de Godzilla (number of Powerfoods: 5)

½   pound extra-lean ground beef or ground turkey

½   cup onion, chopped

2   cloves garlic, minced

½   cup canned kidney beans, rinsed and mashed

2   green chile peppers, seeded and diced

2   teaspoons chili powder

4   large whole-wheat tortillas

⅔   cup shredded lettuce

1   cup chopped tomatoes

½   cup grated low-fat Monterey Jack cheese

1. In a large nonstick skillet over medium-high heat, cook the beef, onion, and garlic until the beef is browned. Drain the fat.

2. Stir in the beans, peppers, and chili powder and cook until hot. Remove from the heat.

3. Warm the tortillas in the microwave for 20 seconds, then fill each with half the mixture. Top with the lettuce, tomatoes, and cheese and roll each tortilla tightly into a tube.

Makes 4 servings

Calories per serving: 270; Protein: 21 g; Carbs: 32 g; Total fat: 9 g; Saturated fat: 4 g; Sodium: 341 mg; Fiber: 6 g

Gone Fishing (number of Powerfoods: 5)

1   tablespoon + 1 teaspoon olive oil

1   trout fillet

1   tablespoon cornmeal

Salt and pepper

½   teaspoon chopped fresh parsley

1   cup French green beans, trimmed and cut into bite-size pieces

2   teaspoons sliced almonds

1. Heat 1 tablespoon of the oil in a nonstick skillet over medium heat.

2. While the pan is heating, sprinkle the flesh side of the trout with the cornmeal, salt, and pepper, pressing lightly so the cornmeal sticks.

3. Place in the pan, flesh side down, and sauté for 4 minutes. Flip and cook for another 2 minutes. Top with the parsley.

4. Place the beans into a steamer basket and steam for 5 minutes. Toss with the remaining 1 teaspoon oil, almonds, salt, and pepper.

Makes 1 serving

Calories per serving: 372; Protein: 20 g; Carbs: 17 g; Total fat: 26 g; Saturated fat: 4 g; Sodium: 48 mg; Fiber: 5 g

Terra Ricotta (number of Powerfoods: 3)

3 tablespoons reduced-fat ricotta cheese

1 teaspoon ready-made roasted garlic

1 ready-made flatbread, such as Flat Out

¾ cup chopped precooked chicken

3 tablespoons grated reduced-fat mozzarella cheese

Salt and pepper

Stir together the ricotta and garlic, blending well. Spread on the flatbread. Top with the chicken and mozzarella. Season to taste with salt and pepper. Bake at 375°F for 6 minutes.

Makes 1 serving

Calories per serving: 352; Protein: 41 g; Carbs: 19 g; Total fat: 13 g; Saturated fat: 6 g; Sodium: 409 mg; Fiber: 2 g

Colonel Mustard (number of Powerfoods: 3)

1 tablespoon maple syrup

1 tablespoon Dijon mustard

1 teaspoon olive oil

Salt and pepper

2 thin-cut boneless pork chops

2 cups Italian salad greens

1 tablespoon low-fat balsamic vinaigrette

1. In a small bowl, stir together the syrup, mustard, oil, salt, and pepper until well blended.

2. Place the chops and mustard mixture inside a large zip-top plastic bag, then shake to coat the chops.

3. Place the chops on a nonstick skillet heated to medium-high, cooking 2 to 3 minutes per side. In the last minute of cooking, pour the remaining mustard mixture onto the chops as they cook.

4. Toss the greens and dressing in a large bowl to coat.

Makes 1 serving

Calories per serving: 393; Protein: 42 g; Carbs: 23 g; Total fat: 17 g; Saturated fat: 5 g; Sodium: 650 mg; Fiber: 2 g

The Orange and Gold (number of Powerfoods: 5)

2	teaspoons peanut oil	⅓	cup chopped celery
¼	teaspoon red-pepper flakes	1	green onion, sliced
2	thin-cut boneless, skinless chicken breasts, cut into bite-size pieces or strips	2	tablespoons chopped unsalted roasted peanuts
⅓	cup matchstick carrots	1	tablespoon hoisin sauce

1. Combine the oil and pepper flakes in a medium-hot skillet.

2. Add the chicken and cook for 2 to 3 minutes, stirring frequently.

3. Add the remaining ingredients and cook for 2 to 3 minutes, stirring frequently. Serve over brown rice.

Makes 1 serving

Calories per serving: 356; Protein: 45 g; Carbs: 18 g; Total fat: 11 g; Saturated fat: 2 g; Sodium: 444 mg; Fiber: 5 g

Chicken Little Italy (number of Powerfoods: 3)

1	tablespoon + 1 teaspoon olive oil	Salt and pepper to taste
1	boneless, skinless chicken breast	¼ cup spaghetti sauce
1	tablespoon Italian-seasoned bread crumbs	1 small clove garlic, crushed
1	teaspoon Parmesan cheese	3 handfuls baby spinach leaves

1. Heat 1 tablespoon of the oil in a nonstick skillet over medium heat.

2. While the pan is heating, pound the chicken to ¼" thickness, then sprinkle with the bread crumbs, cheese, salt, and pepper, pressing lightly so the crumbs stick.

3. Place in the pan and sauté for 2 to 3 minutes per side. Top with nuked spaghetti sauce.

4. Combine the remaining 1 teaspoon oil and the garlic in another nonstick skillet over medium-high heat.

5. Add the spinach, turning frequently with tongs until wilted (about 6 minutes).

Makes 1 serving

Calories per serving: 395; Protein: 32 g; Carbs: 19 g; Total fat: 22 g; Saturated fat: 3 g; Sodium: 608 mg; Fiber: 5 g

Shrimp to Nuts (number of Powerfoods: 4)

2	teaspoons peanut oil	2	teaspoons reduced-sodium soy sauce
¼	teaspoon red-pepper flakes		
½	cup French green beans, cut into bite-size pieces	2	teaspoons orange juice
		¼	teaspoon orange zest
⅓	cup matchstick carrots	1½	cups medium frozen shrimp, defrosted with tails removed
¼	cup whole unsalted roasted cashews		

1. Combine the oil and pepper flakes in a medium-hot skillet.

2. Add everything but the shrimp (they're already precooked before freezing). Cook for 2 to 3 minutes, stirring frequently.

3. Add the shrimp and cook for another 2 to 3 minutes, stirring frequently. Serve over brown rice.

Makes 2 servings

Calories per serving: 332; Protein: 39 g; Carbs: 11 g; Total fat: 15 g; Saturated fat: 3 g; Sodium: 578 mg; Fiber: 2 g

Abs Diet Snacks

MOST DIET PLANS portray snacking as a failure. I want you to think of snacking as exactly the opposite—as a key to success! But the secret to effective snacking is doing so at the optimum time—about 2 hours before you're scheduled to eat your next meal. That'll be enough time to head off hunger pangs and keep you full enough to avoid a meltdown at meal-time. You have a lot of flexibility in what you use to snack. You could use one of the recipes that follow or have a portion of leftovers from dinner, a sandwich, a smoothie, or a combination of some of the Abs Diet Power-foods. To make it easier, turn the page and pick one food from column A and one from column B. That will ensure your satiety.

A		B	
PROTEIN	**DAIRY**	**FRUIT OR VEGETABLE**	**COMPLEX CARBOHYDRATE**
2 teaspoons reduced-fat peanut butter	8 ounces low-fat yogurt	1 ounce raisins	1 or 2 slices whole-grain bread
1 ounce almonds	1 cup 1 percent milk or chocolate milk	Raw vegetables (celery, baby carrots, broccoli), unlimited	1 bowl oatmeal or high-fiber cereal
3 slices low-sodium deli turkey breast	¾ cup low-fat ice cream	1½ cup berries	
3 slices deli roast beef	1½ slices fat-free cheese	4 ounces cantaloupe	
	1 stick string cheese	1 large orange	
		1 can (11.5 ounces) low-sodium V8 juice	

Cucumber Tubes (number of Powerfoods: 5)

- 1 cucumber
- 1 teaspoon finely chopped parsley
- ¼ teaspoon finely chopped basil
- ½ teaspoon finely chopped chives
- ¾ cup low-fat, low-sodium cottage cheese

Cut the cucumber in half lengthwise. Hollow the center of each half by scooping out the seeds with a spoon or vegetable knife. Stir the herbs into the cottage cheese, then arrange in the hollowed cucumbers.

Makes 2 servings

Calories per serving: 84; Protein: 12 g; Carbs: 7 g; Total fat: 1 g; Saturated fat: 1 g; Sodium: 11 mg; Fiber: 2 g

PB Power Apples (number of Powerfoods: 2)

2 tablespoons peanut butter

Dash of cinnamon

1 medium red apple, such as Gala or Red Delicious, halved and cored

In a small bowl, stir together the peanut butter and cinnamon (start with a dash—cinnamon is potent stuff). Spread on each apple half.

Makes 1 serving

Calories per serving: 276; Protein: 8 g; Carbs: 30 g; Total fat: 17 g; Saturated fat: 3 g; Sodium: 1 mg; Fiber: 8 g

Spread Yourself Thin (number of Powerfoods: 2)

1 can (15 ounces) cannellini beans, rinsed and drained

1 tablespoon chopped fresh rosemary

1 clove garlic, crushed

½ lemon, juiced

2 tablespoons olive oil

Salt and pepper

In a blender or food processor, mix the beans, rosemary, garlic, and lemon juice. (If you're using a blender, you may need to stop and scrape the sides of the canister once to make sure everything blends well.) Stream the oil through the top until you reach the desired consistency. Season to taste with salt and pepper.

Calories per 1-tablespoon serving: 21; Protein: 1 g; Carbs: 2 g; Total fat: 1 g; Saturated fat: 0 g; Sodium: 20 mg sodium; Fiber: 1 g

Yogi Pops (number of Powerfoods: 1)

1 6-pack (4-ounce cups) of your favorite flavor of reduced-fat yogurt

6 Popsicle sticks

Pierce each yogurt pack with a stick. Freeze.

Serves 6

Calories per serving: 118; Protein: 4 g; Carbs: 24 g; Total fat: 1 g; Saturated fat: 0 g; Sodium: 59 mg; Fiber: 0 g

Chapter 10

ABS DIET MEAL PLANS
Featuring 3 Perfect Weeks of Eating for Women

NLIKE MOST DIET PLANS, WHICH ARE LADEN with complex, hard-to-follow rules and verboten foods you love but have to live without, the Abs Diet lets you eat the foods you love, keeps your cravings at bay, and helps you control stress—all at the same time. Here's an example of how you can structure a week of eating. It's not written in stone, by any means: Mix up the meals. Substitute whenever you want. Heck, I don't care if you eat the same thing every day for a week. The purpose of these sample weeks are simply to show you how to follow the principles of the Abs Diet. So enjoy!

The calories in the weekly meal plans below are tailored to provide between 1,400 and 1,600 calories per day. But every woman has different caloric needs, depending on her current weight and activity level (page 65 gave you a formula to figure out yours). Use these weekly meal plans as a base, but you can also adjust either up or down. If you want to reduce your calories, don't skip a meal—remember, eating six times a day helps keep your metabolism moving. Instead, cut the portion size of a regular meal or eliminate part of a snack. If your formula shows that you should add calories, I recommend that you increase in small ways, such as drinking a few more ounces of smoothie for a meal or snack or adding a handful of nuts at a snack, rather than augmenting too much during your meals, where there's more chance of doling out larger-than-you-need portions.

Perfect Week, Sample 1

MONDAY: 1,443 CALORIES

Breakfast

Change Your Tuna (page 117)

Snack #1

8 ounces Belly-Busting Berry smoothie (page 112), 1 apple

Lunch

Crunch Time (page 122), 1 stick string cheese

Snack #2

Cucumber Tubes (page 136)

Dinner

Gone Fishing (page 132)

Snack #3

Low-fat ice cream sandwich

TUESDAY: 1,568 CALORIES

Breakfast

Mint Condition (page 117)

Snack #1

8 ounces Show Me the Honey smoothie (page 113)

FIVE WAYS TO ADD MORE FIBER

To your eggs: A third of a cup of chopped onion and a clove of garlic will add 1 gram of fiber to a couple of scrambled eggs.

To your sandwich: Hate whole wheat? Go with rye. Like wheat, it has 2 grams of fiber per slice. That's more than twice the amount of fiber in white.

To your dinner: Have a sweet potato. It has 2 grams more fiber than a typical Idaho potato.

To your cereal: Half a cup of raspberries adds 4 grams of fiber.

To your snack: Eat trail mix. Half a cup of raisin bran, 1 ounce of mixed nuts, and five dried apricot halves give you almost 7 grams of fiber.

Lunch

Roll of a Lifetime (page 124), 1 cup berries

Snack #2

1 stick string cheese, 5 to 7 whole-wheat crackers, such as Triscuits

Dinner

Terra Ricotta (page 133)

Snack #3

Yogi Pops (page 137)

WEDNESDAY: 1,407 CALORIES

Breakfast

Mo' Feta, Mo' Betta (page 117)

Snack #1

8 ounces Extreme Chocolate smoothie (page 113)

Lunch

Popeye and Olive Oil (page 124)

Snack #2

½ PB Power Apples (page 137)

Dinner

Colonel Mustard (page 133)

Snack #3

Low-fat ice cream sandwich

THURSDAY: 1,510 CALORIES

Breakfast

Waffles Rancheros (page 118), 1 pear

Snack #1

8 ounces Pumpkin You Up! smoothie (page 113)

Lunch

Reuben Reduced (page 125)

Snack #2

1 stick string cheese, 5 to 7 whole-wheat crackers, such as Triscuits

Dinner

The Orange and Gold (page 134)

Snack #3

Yogi Pops (page 137)

FRIDAY: 1,490 CALORIES

Breakfast

Breakfast with Barbie (page 118)

Snack #1

8 ounces Coco Poof smoothie (page 114)

Lunch

The Melon Banquet (page 125)

Snack #2

Cucumber Tubes (page 136)

Dinner

Chicken Little Italy (page 134)

Snack #3

1 carton low-fat yogurt with fruit

SATURDAY: 1,424 CALORIES

Breakfast

Corn to Be Wild (page 118), 1 orange

Snack #1

8 ounces Belly-Busting Berry smoothie (page 112)

Lunch

The Two Chicks (page 125)

Snack #2

2 tablespoons Spread Yourself Thin (page 137), ¾ cup broccoli or carrots

Dinner

Shrimp to Nuts (page 135)

Snack #3

Yogi Pops (page 137)

SUNDAY: 1,294 CALORIES PLUS CHEAT MEAL

Breakfast

The 'Bama Bowl (page 119), ½ cup orange juice

Snack #1

4 ounces Lemon Drips and Drops smoothie (page 114)

Lunch

Pimp My Shrimp (page 126)

Snack

4 to 8 ounces Lemon Drips and Drops smoothie,
1 cup melon

Dinner

Cheat meal

Perfect Week, Sample 2

MONDAY: 1,457 CALORIES

Breakfast

One glass (8 ounces) Abs Diet Ultimate Power Smoothie
(page 110); make extra for later

Snack #1

1 teaspoon peanut butter, raw vegetables (as much as you
want)

Lunch

Turkey or roast beef sandwich on whole-grain bread, 1 cup
1 percent or fat-free milk, 1 apple

Snack #2

1 ounce almonds, 1½ cups berries

Dinner

Italian Chowin' (page 126)

Snack #3

4 ounces Abs Diet Ultimate Power Smoothie

TUESDAY: 1,472 CALORIES

Breakfast

Eggs Beneficial Sandwich (page 115), 1 cup fat-free milk

Snack #1

1 teaspoon peanut butter, 1 bowl oatmeal or high-fiber cereal

Lunch

The I-Am-Not-Eating-Salad Salad (page 120)

Snack #2

3 slices deli turkey, 1 large orange

Dinner

Brazilian Chicken (page 127)

Snack #3

1 ounce almonds, 4 ounces cantaloupe

WEDNESDAY: 1,578 CALORIES

Breakfast

One glass (8 ounces) Strawberry Field Marshall Smoothie (page 110); make extra for later

Snack #1

1 ounce raisins

Lunch

Guac and Roll (page 121)

Snack #2

1 stick string cheese, raw vegetables (as much as you want)

Dinner

Chile-Peppered Steak (page 128)

Snack #3

4 to 8 ounces Strawberry Field Marshall Smoothie

THURSDAY: 1,564 CALORIES

Breakfast

1 slice whole-grain bread with 1 teaspoon peanut butter, ½ cup All-Bran cereal with 1 cup 1 percent or fat-free milk, 1 cup berries

Snack #1

8 ounces low-fat yogurt, 1 can low-sodium V8 juice

Lunch

Guilt-Free BLT (page 120)

Snack #2

3 slices lean deli roast beef, 1 large orange

Dinner

Easy Cheesy (page 128)

Snack #3

1 teaspoon peanut butter, ½ cup low-fat ice cream

FRIDAY: 1,584 CALORIES

Breakfast

One glass (8 ounces) Banana Split Smoothie (page 111); make extra for later

Snack #1

1 ounce almonds, 4 ounces cantaloupe

Lunch

Hot Tuna (page 121)

Snack #2

3 slices lean deli roast beef, 1 large orange

Dinner

Chili Con Turkey (page 129)

Snack #3

4 ounces Banana Split Smoothie

SATURDAY: 1,071 CALORIES PLUS CHEAT MEAL

Breakfast

One tall glass (8 ounces) Halle Berries Smoothie (page 111); make extra for later

Snack #1

> 1 cup high-fiber cereal, 1 cup low-fat yogurt

Lunch

> Leftover Chili Con Turkey

Snack #2

> 1 teaspoon peanut butter, 1 or 2 slices whole-grain bread

Dinner

> Cheat meal! Have whatever you've been craving this week: wine and cheese, burgers, fillet of whatever—anything you can dream of.

Snack #3

> 4 ounces Halle Berries Smoothie

HOW TO PICK PRODUCE

A lot of us grew up with an aversion to fruits and vegetables, mostly caused by doting parents who boiled canned greens into pulp and then insisted that by not eating them, we were somehow responsible for kids in China not having enough rice. Today, you've got one way to prove your parents wrong: by showing them how really delicious fresh produce can be, if you know how to pick it and prepare it.

Berries. Before you buy raspberries or strawberries, flip the carton over. You're looking for nature's expiration date: juice stains. You want berries you can eat without looking like you've been fingerprinted.

Watermelon. Forget color, shape, or size: Watermelons are best judged by weight. The heavier a melon is, the more water it contains, and water is what helps give a melon its flavor.

Cantaloupe. Don't knock on a melon to check its ripeness; slap it instead. You're listening for a hollow ring, not a dull thud or an inhuman scream.

Tomatoes. Look for tomatoes that are firm and heavy for their size. They should have a sweet tomato aroma. If you generally don't like tomatoes, try the yellow kind; they tend to have a sweeter, less acidic flavor than red varieties.

Peaches. Look for well-colored fruit with no green spots. The flesh should yield slightly when lightly pressed and should have a fragrant aroma. (Fragrant like a peach, not fragrant like your cousin Freddy.)

SUNDAY: 1,579 CALORIES

Breakfast

The I-Haven't-Had-My-Coffee-Yet Sandwich (page 116)

Snack #1

1 teaspoon peanut butter, 1 can low-sodium V8 juice

Brunch (relax—it's Sunday):

2 scrambled eggs, 2 slices whole-grain toast, 1 banana,
1 cup 1 percent or fat-free milk

Snack #2

2 slices lean deli roast beef, 1 slice fat-free cheese

Dinner

BBQ King (page 130)

Snack #3

1 ounce almonds, ½ cup low-fat ice cream

Perfect Week, Sample 3

MONDAY: 1,592 CALORIES

Breakfast

3-egg-white omelet with chopped vegetables, 1 whole-
wheat English muffin with 2 teaspoons soft margarine

Snack #1

Raw mixed vegetables, ¼ cup hummus

Lunch

3 ounces sliced turkey breast in a whole-wheat tortilla with
mixed greens, tomato, and 2 or 3 slices of avocado;
1 cup mixed green salad with 2 teaspoons olive oil and
vinegar

Snack #2

1 cup berries mixed with 2 tablespoons fat-free plain
yogurt

Dinner

Asian chicken salad: 2 cups mixed greens, red onions, and
tomato wedges; 3 ounces cooked chicken breast, sliced;

½ cup mandarin orange sections; and 1 ounce cashews tossed with 1 tablespoon olive oil and vinegar; 4 whole-grain crackers

Snack #3

1 piece fruit, 1 cup fat-free plain or artificially sweetened yogurt

TUESDAY: 1,597 CALORIES

Breakfast

1 cup whole-grain cereal with 2 tablespoons raisins and 1 cup fat-free or 1 percent milk, 1 banana

Snack #1

1 container fat-free plain yogurt mixed with 2 tablespoons dried fruit and 2 teaspoons honey

Lunch

1 cup broth-based or tomato soup; 2 ounces sliced lean roast beef with lettuce, tomato, and mustard on 2 slices of whole-wheat bread

Snack #2

1 stick string cheese, 2 whole-wheat crackers

Dinner

1 cup cooked white or brown rice, 3 ounces grilled shrimp in gumbo sauce, mixed green salad with 2 teaspoons olive oil and vinegar

Snack #3

1 large whole-wheat pretzel

WEDNESDAY: 1,427 CALORIES

Breakfast

1 cup oatmeal with 2 tablespoons mixed dried fruit and nuts and 1 teaspoon cinnamon, ¼ cup fat-free plain yogurt, 1 cup orange or grapefruit juice

Snack #1

¼ cup microwave air-popped popcorn (100 calories' worth; see package)

Lunch

tuna salad: 3 ounces grilled or canned tuna, 5 small red potatoes, ½ cup string beans, and 5 to 8 olives on a bed of salad greens tossed with 2 teaspoons olive oil and 1 tablespoon red-wine vinegar

Snack #2

1 large rectangular graham cracker with 1 teaspoon nut butter, 1 piece fruit

Dinner

1 vegetarian burger with lettuce, tomato, and red onion on a soft wheat roll; side salad of mixed greens and vegetables and 2 teaspoons olive oil and vinegar dressing

Snack #3

½ cup fat-free ice cream or frozen yogurt

THURSDAY: 1,564 CALORIES

Breakfast

¾ cup muesli with 1 cup fat-free milk, 1 orange or ½ grapefruit

Snack #1

1 ounce low-fat cheese, 2 whole-wheat crackers

Lunch

tossed salad: mixed salad greens, cucumber, red bell pepper, red onion, diced carrots, tomato, ½ cup chickpeas, ½ cup string beans, and 1 ounce grated hard cheese tossed with 2 teaspoons olive oil and 1 tablespoon red-wine vinegar; 1 small whole-wheat roll

Snack #2

1 cup fortified soy milk, 2 Whole Grain Fig Newton cookies

Dinner

spaghetti marinara: 1 cup cooked whole-grain pasta topped with ½ cup marinara sauce and 1 tablespoon grated Romano cheese, side salad with olive oil and vinegar or light dressing

Snack #3

2 kiwifruits

FRIDAY: 1,115 CALORIES PLUS CHEAT MEAL

Breakfast

1 cup hot oatmeal with ¼ cup fat-free plain yogurt and
2 tablespoons raisins

Snack #1

1 energy bar like a PowerBar Pria or a Luna bar

Lunch

2 ounces whole-wheat pita, 2 ounces chicken or turkey
breast, 1 tablespoon cranberry sauce with chopped mixed
greens

Snack #2

1 container fat-free fruit-flavored yogurt with banana

Dinner

Cheat meal

Snack #3

1 low-fat or fat-free brownie, 1 cup fat-free milk

SATURDAY: 1,557 CALORIES

Breakfast

2 eggs and 1 egg white, scrambled; 2 slices whole-wheat
toast with 2 teaspoons soft margarine and 1 tablespoon
jam; ½ cup mixed fruit and ½ cup fat-free yogurt

Snack #1

½ whole-wheat pita with 1 tablespoon hummus

Lunch

1 cup chicken noodle soup, 4 whole-wheat crackers, mixed
green salad with 1 tablespoon grated hard cheese and 5
sliced olives tossed with 2 teaspoons olive oil and vinegar

Snack #2

1½ cups watermelon chunks

Dinner

4 ounces broiled lean steak, ½ cup mashed potatoes
(made with soft margarine), 1 cup steamed broccoli with
2 teaspoons Parmesan cheese

Snack #3

1 piece fresh fruit with ½ cup sorbet

SUNDAY: 1,448 CALORIES

Breakfast

2 whole-wheat frozen toaster waffles topped with
1 tablespoon nut butter and ½ medium banana, sliced;
1 cup fat-free milk

Snack #1

8 ounces low-fat yogurt

Lunch

1 medium baked potato topped with sautéed mixed
vegetables (e.g., mushrooms, onions, broccoli) in
1 tablespoon olive oil with 1 ounce grated hard cheese

Snack #2

10 almonds or cashews

Dinner

turkey or chicken burger: 4 ounces grilled or broiled
chicken or turkey (white meat only) with onions, tomatoes,
and lettuce on whole-wheat roll; mixed greens tossed with
2 teaspoons olive oil and vinegar

Snack #3

1 4-ounce fat-free pudding

Chapter **11**

ABS DIET ADAPTATIONS
Tailoring the Plan for Each Woman's Individual Needs

THE ROADBLOCK TO ANY SUCCESSFUL WEIGHT-LOSS PLAN is clearly marked with a capital I: Inconvenience. If a diet doesn't fit into your work hours, your lifestyle, your health, or your habits, then it's going to fail faster than a Rob Schneider movie. Going to Subway for virtually every meal isn't convenient for most people, nor is cooking up a pound of bacon every morning for breakfast, nor is asking the server at a restaurant to pop a frozen dinner into the microwave and nuke it for 3 minutes. A lot of diets simply aren't that convenient to follow. I believe that the Abs Diet is convenient—because it gives you enough guidelines to help you understand what healthy eating is while also giving you enough flexibility to make it work for you whether you eat at home, out, in the car, or while watching your kids' soccer and ballet practices.

That said, sticking to a diet—or, rather, changing your eating lifestyle—isn't just a matter of how it fits into your schedule but also how it fits into your life and into your body. Women's needs may be a little different than those of the typical guy—namely, you're likely a little more tuned in to your health than he is, and there are certain biological fundamentals that make your body different than his (more on hormones and pregnancy in later chapters). And that's why I want to outline some strategies that may be of help to women in particular—based on feed-back I've heard from women about what they want in addition to the fundamental principles, strategies, and recipes of the Abs Diet.

So, here, I'd like to outline some of the things you can do to make the six major Abs Diet principles work to complement your life, your personality, and your health—and not compete against them.

If You're a Calorie Counter . . .

PERSONALLY, I'D RATHER watch aforementioned Rob Schneider movies than count calories—too tedious a job and too inexact a science if you're eating on the run. But I also realize that many of you like to count calories for a couple of reasons: Mainly, doing so can really help give you a fairly accurate gauge of whether you're staying in your optimum caloric range (especially because your caloric requirements are lower than men's and because all of us tend to miscalculate portion sizes). In the major Abs Diet guidelines I laid out in Chapter 7, I explained that eating Powerfoods is really one way to let the foods count calories for you—if you eat a balance of good, healthy foods six times a day. That doesn't mean that you can't count calories if that works best with your personality. So if you're going to be a calorie counter, you need to arm yourself with three tools to help make counting as manageable as possible.

1. **A food diary.** Write down everything you eat and drink as you consume it. The only way to accurately tally is to keep a running list, rather than trying to remember at the end of the day.

2. **Measuring cups and food scales.** The fact is, most of us underestimate the amount of food we actually eat (thanks, in large part, to restaurants that serve about 133 serving sizes in one dinner entrée). After a few weeks of measuring out cereal and weighing your fish, you'll be much better at eyeballing and dividing up accurate serving and portion sizes.

3. **A comprehensive listing of calories,** so you can quickly find what you need. Luckily, this one's easy. Yours begins on page 359.

Some other things to think about if you're going to include calorie tallying as part of the Abs Diet:

Estimate your caloric needs. As evidenced by cars and super-models, not everything is built in the same way. To figure out how many calories you need to maintain your current weight, multiply your weight in pounds by 11 and add 200 to 300 if you exercise regularly. For example, a sedentary 155-pound woman needs about 1,705 calories a day; an active one might need 2,005. (For a more detailed formula that's tailored to your body, flip back to page 65.) Then decide how fast you want to lose the weight. A pound of body weight equals 3,500 calories, so you would need to shave 500 a day from your count to drop a pound a week. The

WHAT'S A 100-CALORIE PORTION?

Proteins

2 ounces or 2 slices low-fat American or Cheddar cheese

2 slices bacon

2 ounces chicken (no skin)

2 small eggs

1½ cups fat-free milk

1 cup 1-percent milk

½ ounce roasted peanuts

2 ounces pork

2 ounces salmon or tuna

4 ounces (about 15) shrimp

Fats

1 tablespoon butter

2 teaspoons olive or corn oil

1 tablespoon mayo

1 tablespoon peanut butter

Carbs

¾ cup All-Bran cereal

1 large apple

1 medium banana

2 cups (about 50) green beans

½ cup corn

¾ cup plain oatmeal

1 ounce pasta

½ medium baked potato

20 medium strawberries

8 teaspoons sugar

2½ slices low-calorie wheat bread

best balance, according to a review of studies on diet composition in the *Journal of the American Dietetic Association*, is 35 to 50 percent carbs, 25 to 35 percent fat, and about 25 to 30 percent protein.

Fiber up. If you're making every calorie count, your best play is to make sure you're going heavy on the high-fiber foods. That's because foods rich in water and fiber are bulkier but less caloric. A cup of strawberries, for example, has about the same calorie content as a small cookie but is far more satisfying. In one study at Pennsylvania State University, women ate the same weight of food over a 2-day period. When the women ate higher-fiber foods on the second day, they took in 30 percent fewer calories but didn't feel any hungrier or less full.

Stick to the six. A British study found that women who ate the same number of meals every day ate fewer calories than those who changed it up from day to day and sometimes skipped breakfast or worked through lunch or ate dessert and then a late-night snack. Plus, when the women ate inconsistently, their metabolisms slowed.

Get to know your servings. Most portion sizes from restaurants and take-out places are well beyond an acceptable serving size. You need to start thinking that those dishes are two (or three) meals instead of one. Also, when you cook meals, serve them up on small plates: Less food will look like more, and you'll eat less.

Don't fear the frozens. Not all frozen foods are the nutritional equivalent of the boxes they come in. Some are healthy (find ones with low trans fats, saturated fats, sugars, and high-fructose corn syrup). The best part is that they enforce a calorie ceiling on you. A study in the *International Journal of Obesity* showed that people who regularly use meal replacements like Slim-Fast and Healthy Choice lose nearly twice as much weight as those on a low-calorie diet. Why? Because those meals have preset portions and a controlled number of calories.

Know the most satisfying foods. In what seems to be a bit of voodoo math, one calorie doesn't always equal one calorie—because of the effect that foods have on how much you want to eat later. Australian researchers developed a satiety index to determine how satisfied you feel after eating. Study participants ate a 240-calorie portion of each food, then rated their satiety over 2 hours. These are the most satisfying foods (notice how many Powerfoods made the list!), so they help you control hunger and decrease your calories during the day.

White potatoes	Fish	Beef
Eggs	Soup	Salad
Oatmeal	Apples	Popcorn
Beans		

If You're a Vegetarian . . .

BEING A VEGETARIAN has a lot of benefits besides never having to endure the 2-hour wait for a table at the popular steak joint. Not only do vegetarians who eat dairy products and eggs typically get their essential vitamins and minerals but—not surprisingly—research also finds that vegetarians typically eat more nutrient-rich fruits, vegetables, legumes, nuts, and whole grains than meat-eaters do. They also tend to eat less fat, including unhealthy saturated fat, and are less likely to be overweight. Because many of the Abs Diet Powerfoods are vegetarian-friendly, you can follow the same principles I've outlined, so long as you keep in mind some special considerations.

Get enough protein. Because you won't be getting your all-important protein in the form of lean meats, make sure you get at least three daily servings of protein-packed, low-fat dairy products such as milk and yogurt (in addition to cheese), as well as two to three eggs per week. When scientists from McMaster University in Ontario assessed the food intake of 617 dieters, they found that eating more protein can reduce the amount of fat around your midsection. Specifically, people who consumed an average of 20 grams of extra protein per day lowered their waist-to-hip ratio measurements by 24 percent, compared with dieters who ate more carbs.

Go nuts. Nuts are also good sources of protein, healthy fats, vitamins, and minerals. Walnuts, canola oil, and flaxseed can replace fish because they are good sources of heart-healthy omega-3 fatty acids.

Savor the soy. The good part about skipping meat is that you're also skipping the cuts that have more blubber than a Sea World tank. The FDA recommends getting at least 25 grams of soy protein each day (for its cardiovascular and other health benefits). It's easy to get, too: 8 ounces of soy milk contains 8 grams of soy protein, one soy burger contains 10 grams, and ¼ cup of soy nuts contains 12 grams. Another option: Green vegetable soybeans (edamame) make a healthy, satisfying snack.

Take your vitamins. A German study found levels of vitamin B_{12} low enough to cause attention, mood, and thinking problems in 68 percent of vegetarians and low enough to raise blood homocysteine (a risk factor for heart disease, dementia, and Alzheimer's) in 38 percent. Remedy: a daily multivitamin with 100 percent of the daily value for B_{12} (6 micrograms).

Pump some dietary iron. Only 2 to 10 percent of the iron in plants is absorbed by your digestive tract, so drink a glass of high–vitamin C juice (citrus or tomato) at the same meal as high-iron foods such as beans, because vitamin C can unlock iron from plants.

Remember, you don't have license to gorge. Just because you're not eating fatty cuts of meat doesn't mean you can make an all-out food fest of chips, bread, baked goods, cookies, crackers, and sweets that are allowed on vegetarian diets.

If You're Lactose Intolerant . . .

IF YOUR BODY CAN'T digest the sugar that's in milk, it's likely that those darn milk mustaches aren't the only things that disturb you. You're probably looking at the dairy products (and their amazing benefits) on the list of Powerfoods and wondering if there's another way you can get those same benefits.

It's true that people who are lactose intolerant don't typically get enough calcium (about 700 milligrams a day, compared with the 1,200 that are recommended for healthy bones). And that can be a problem: Besides the bone-building benefits of calcium, you also want it for the effects it seems to have on weight loss. If dairy leaves you gassy, crampy, and bloated, you can avoid a calcium deficit in these ways.

▶ Drink milk made for people with lactose intolerance, such as Lactaid.

▶ Try yogurt; the enzymes it contains digest milk sugar for you.

▶ Take a calcium supplement, plus 400 IU of vitamin D.

▶ Eat nondairy foods that have lots of calcium, such as sardines, almonds, and broccoli.

▶ Snack on Cheddar or Swiss cheese—two naturally low-lactose cheeses.

If You've Got IBS . . .

I KNOW IT SOUNDS like a government agency or a new TV station, but IBS (irritable bowel syndrome) is something that disturbs 50 million Americans—about 75 percent of whom are women, according to the US Department of Health and Human Services. In normal digestion, the walls of your intestines contract and then relax as they transport food from your stomach. When you have IBS, the contractions are stronger and longer, causing diarrhea, constipation, or bouts of both. It's not clear why women are so disproportionately affected by the condition, but researchers suspect it may be related to hormone fluctuations throughout the menstrual cycle. In any case, here's what you can do to help with the pain.

▶ Eating your six smaller meals a day will help naturally by keeping you from overloading your digestive tract with larger amounts of food three times a day.

▶ Limit your consumption of fructose, a sugar found in fruits and most refined foods. Research shows that fructose is related to more severe symptoms of IBS.

▶ Keep a journal to track which foods cause the most discomfort. Researchers at St. George's Hospital in London analyzed blood samples from 108 IBS patients and 43 healthy folks to check their reactions to 16 foods, including nuts, meat, dairy, and grains.

More severe reactions were triggered by wheat, beef, pork, and lamb. Surprisingly, dairy products—a group anecdotally linked to IBS—caused no problems. If you have IBS, cut back on meat and wheat, and keep a diary to pinpoint which foods cause distress.

▶ The herb peppermint relaxes the digestive tract's smooth muscles, easing spasms. German research found that capsules containing 180 to 200 milligrams of peppermint oil eased IBS pain, bloating, and gas for 58 percent of takers. Look for capsules with an enteric coating that helps prevent them from causing heartburn. Take one with a glass of water before dinner.

▶ Make sure to stick to your workouts. Physical activity helps regulate those intestinal contractions. A University of Washington study found that those people with IBS who exercised regularly had fewer symptoms than those who didn't.

If You're On Antidepressants . . .

THESE DAYS, antidepressants seem almost as prevalent as iPods. Doctors prescribe them for a number of reasons, including depression, libido issues, and smoking cessation. While some antidepressants are weight neutral, others (like classes of drugs called SSRIs) can actually make you gain weight. Talk to your doctor about getting a new drug with the same antidepressant effect but without the weight gain. One medication that seems to even have a weight-loss effect is Bupropion. In a study of 422 overweight people, those taking Bupropion lost nearly 10 pounds, while those on a placebo lost about 3½ pounds.

If You're Likely to Give In to Temptation . . .

HOWEVER YOU SPEND your days—whether you work out of the house, whether you work in the house, whether you're running a business, or whether you're running a household—I have no doubt that you're multitasking. You're trying to get kids here and there, trying to advance your career, and reeling from all the technology that's supposed to make our lives easier. (How much chocolate did you down the last time your computer crashed?) The effect: We're under the gun. All the time. Sometimes, the only solace we can get from the rigors of life is in the refrigerator. And that, my friends, is clinically classified as Not Good. Here's how to deal with some of the stresses and temptations in life so that you don't make your waist pay the price for your stress.

Working late in the office: Keep fiber-rich snacks such as Country Choice's Oatmeal Squares or Luna bars in your desk drawer. Fiber, as opposed to an instant sugar rush, takes more time to release glucose into your bloodstream. This will keep you energized and full longer, plus improve brain function and productivity.

Feeding the kids: It may be tempting to snort up the last 10 fries or scoop out a few spoonfuls of SpaghettiOs, but they're just going to add on extra calories without nutrients. Anything your kid doesn't finish (and can't eat later) should immediately be thrown away so that you don't clean the plate. Also, buy snacks high in calcium, like chocolate milk, low-fat yogurt, or string cheese, so that if you do pick from their plates, at least you're not doing so with Ding Dongs.

Partying with coworkers: Eat an apple and a handful of nuts an hour before you go so you won't feel like gorging on three-story appetizers when you get there.

YOU SNOOZE, YOU LOSE

One of the best ways to lose more weight: Sleep more hours. A study by researchers at Stanford University and the University of Wisconsin found that people who slept less had lower levels of leptin (the hormone that suppresses appetite) and higher levels of ghrelin (the hormone that makes you hungry). Not getting enough shut-eye? Try these strategies.

▶ Set aside a half hour to an hour of "transition time" for a warm bath, gentle yoga, or anything that puts your mind on pause.

▶ Aim for 7 to 9 hours of sleep each night. Record the late-night shows you like, and go to bed at a reasonable time. That'll make it easier to wake up each day when the alarm goes off.

▶ When you do crawl into bed later than usual, don't stay up or sleep in more than 2 hours past normal.

If You're a Believer in the Theory That Little Things Count . . .

IF YOU'RE WORKING with a daily calorie intake of somewhere in the neighborhood of 1,400 to 1,600 calories, then yes, every calorie does count. The following little tricks may not seem like they have a huge effect, but when you add up these changes over a period of time, they'll translate into a leaner and stronger body.

Blot. Use a paper napkin to blot a teaspoon of fat off a pizza slice. At a slice a week, that's more than a whole cup of fat you won't eat—or wear—this year.

Tighten your belt. When you feel a craving and temptation to gorge, tighten your belt a notch—as a reminder of the size you'd like to be.

Get more milk. Consuming 1,800 milligrams of calcium a day could block the absorption of about 80 calories. Fill your coffee mug with skim or 1 percent milk, drink it down to the level you want in your coffee, then pour in your caffeine fix.

Buy cut veggies. They cost more, but they'll pay dividends later—because you're more likely to snack on them than on some other, less healthy food.

Get water down. A recent German study showed that drinking water burns calories. Drinking about 2 cups of cold water—no warmer than 72 degrees—used up roughly 25 calories. Drink a liter a day and you're talking 5 pounds a year.

Go smaller. Use a salad plate instead of a dinner plate. Studies show that putting your portions on smaller dishes means you'll end up eating less at a meal.

Dilute juice. Add water to your fruit juice to reduce calories.

Make your drinks count. Have a V8 or tomato juice instead of a Diet Coke.

Have a Power snack prepared. Mix three different kinds of beans and sprinkle in some low-cal Italian dressing. Have it as a snack all week.

Think about eating. Eat without doing anything else—no TV, no reading, no working.

Stop mindless snacking. Chew a strong-flavored gum like cinnamon while you're cooking. Sneaking a taste of the food will be less appealing.

YOUR PERFECT VITAMIN

Though not every multivitamin/mineral will meet all your nutritional needs, yours should include these nutrients. Clip this list to see how your multi stacks up, or take it with you if you're shopping for a new multi.

NUTRIENT	AMOUNT PER TABLET
Vitamin A	5,000 IU
Beta-carotene	20 percent of vitamin A
Vitamin D	200 IU
Vitamin E	30 IU
Vitamin K	90 mcg
Folic acid	400 mcg
Vitamin B_6	2 mg
Vitamin B_{12}	2.4 mcg
Vitamin C	75 mg
Calcium	1,000 mg
Chromium	25 mcg
Copper	2 mg
Iron	18 mg
Magnesium	400 mg
Omega-3 fats	1 g
Selenium	55 mcg
Zinc	8 mg

WHAT'S ON YOUR MIND?

Psychological Strategies for Dealing with Your Obstacles—And Your Changing Moods

THERE'S A REASON WHY THERE ARE MORE DIET PLANS than there are *American Idol* wannabes: because many of them are pretty darn lousy. Why? Not necessarily because of the food plan and nutritional choices (though there are plenty of those that are lousy), but many times because of all the other stuff that comes with the nutritional nuts and bolts. That is, how does what's happening in your mind affect what's happening in your stomach? How realistic is it to think that you can stick to the diet over the long term? How low maintenance is the actual plan?

I believe that the Abs Diet goes a long way toward eliminating some of the intangible issues that often come with dieting. For example, the once-a-week cheat meal allows you to give in to temptations so you're not constantly denying yourself a hunk of 32-cheese lasagna. The six meals a day keep you from feeling starved and frustrated. And the delicious smoothies satisfy the daily cravings for sweets—a satisfaction that's absent from so many diet plans. That said, I know that anytime you make a change in your approach to eating or exercise, you're going to face more obstacles than a boot-camp recruit. And I believe that much of your success will come not only from following the guidelines and principles of the Abs Diet but also from having some strategies to cope with the psychological aspects of changing the way you eat and the way you exercise.

Struggle 1: Feeling Full versus Feeling Starving

WE'VE BEEN CONDITIONED to believe that the only way we're supposed to feel on a diet is starving, famished, and about 3 seconds away from gnawing on the drywall. Somehow, denying ourselves food makes us feel like we're accomplishing something. But the fact is, the more you starve yourself, the more you slow your metabolism, and the more weight you're going to end up gaining.

On the flip side, you don't want to live your whole life feeling like you just finished Thanksgiving dinner. You shouldn't feel bloated, gross, and ready to pop. The feeling you want is somewhere in the middle—in a state of nutritional satisfaction.

When following the Abs Diet dictum of eating six times a day, that satisfaction is what you should feel. But it may take some time for you to make the adjustment—because you're not used to feeling *satisfied* when you're "on a diet."

One of the best ways to reset your satiety clock is to make sure you don't skimp on breakfast. Researchers in the Netherlands found that those who started the day with a high-calorie meal rich in complex carbohydrates were more likely to feel satisfied for longer. Aim for a breakfast that's 20 percent of your caloric needs for the day (about 350 calories) and full of slow-burning complex carbs. That means a bowl of raisin bran and one slice of whole-wheat toast with all-fruit preserves, or a half cup of multigrain oatmeal and half a sliced banana sprinkled into a small container of low-fat vanilla yogurt. It may take a few weeks to retrain your mind into thinking that staying in a state of satisfaction is good for you. But if you can set your stomach up for a perfect day of eating, you'll have a better shot of doing the same for your mind.

Struggle 2: You're Edgy When You're Just Starting Out

IT'S NO SECRET that going on a diet can be as tough on your mind as it is on your local ice-cream shop: A recent UCLA study linked dieting to chronic stress. Not only can it make you revert to your old eating habits but it can also keep you fat because cortisol, a hormone released during stress, slows down weight loss. This is when you need to rely on your friends for support—or even ask them to join you in your weight-loss crusade. Researchers from the United Kingdom found that women who dieted as part of a group had less stress than those who went it alone.

The good news is that the uncomfortable feeling you experience when you first adjust your eating routine should last only a little while; it takes only 21 days for a repeated action to become a natural habit.

Struggle 3: Your PMS Munchies Have You Craving Cheat Meals More Than Once a Week

DURING THE FINAL 14 days of your menstrual cycle, progesterone is elevated. When that happens, the feel-good hormone serotonin

---

WORKOUT STRUGGLES

We all have times when it's tough to psych ourselves up for our workout routines. Here's a rundown of the most common workout obstacles and the best ways to get past them.

Strength training: So what if it's 8 reps or 12? Whether you're doing crunches, bench presses, or lunges, it's easy to lose motivation when you're doing rep after rep after rep.

The Fix: Keep your eye on your goals. You build strength when your muscles break down and your body repairs them by creating tougher muscle tissue. You barely begin to break down muscles during the first few reps, which is why you need to pick a weight that allows you to complete 10 challenging yet doable reps without compromising form.

Running: Sore legs. If your body is producing lactic acid during one of the interval sessions that you'll learn about on page 208, it can cause a burning decreases, along with endorphins and dopamine, two chemicals responsible for helping your body fight stress. The combination makes your mood plummet and your appetite soar. This is why it's especially important to stick to your six meals. Eating often helps stabilize your blood sugar, cut fatigue, and prevent bloating. You'll find more on combating PMS and other hormone-related eating habits in Chapter 16.

Struggle 4: You're Not Seeing the Scale Move

AFTER ABOUT 6 WEEKS of steady exercise, you'll notice that you have more muscle and less fat—even if the number on the scale hasn't changed. That's because muscle weighs more than fat. So you have to remember that even though your weight might not be dropping, you're still making progress. Your new muscle is helping you burn even more fat because, as you remember, muscle tissue uses more calories than fat cells do. So the more muscle you possess, the more calories you'll burn—even when you're not working out.

Look at other ways to measure your progress besides your scale, such as the way your clothes fit, or an improvement in the amount of

---

sensation in your quads and glutes. That soreness is pain you can push through and a positive indicator of how hard you're working.

The Fix: Resting for a minute or two will allow your body to take in more oxygen, which you need to help flush the lactic acid. Stretch while you rest to separate the muscle fibers and improve circulation. Try the Stork to stretch quads and hips: Stand on one leg and pull the other behind you, bringing your heel toward your butt.

Cardio machines: Boring! Your brain is zoning out, and your body needs new stimulation as it adapts to repetitive movement patterns.

The Fix: All the more reason to make sure your cardio workouts are interval sessions. They'll trick your mind into thinking the workout is moving quicker, and you'll challenge your muscles, burning more calories and building strength. Do 2 minutes at a fast pace, then drop it down for 1 minute, alternating until you're suddenly out of time.

exercise you do, or changes in the size of your body parts. Save the scale for once-a-month measurements if you're easily frustrated by small changes in weight.

Your Mood, Your Meal

THERE ARE A LOT of things that can change your mood for the better—a beautiful sunset, a productive workout, a flirty e-mail sent at the right time by the right person. There are also a lot of things that can do the opposite—a gray sky, a twisted ankle, or a snarky e-mail sent at the wrong time by the wrong person. It's no secret that our moods can swing faster than a 7-year-old at a playground, but one of the tricks for battling out of a bad mood or foul feelings is using nature's medicine—food—to your advantage. By eating the healthy foods that can pick you up, you help your mind—without hurting your body.

When you're blue: The thing you may reach for when you're feeling a little on the weepy side may be the hunk of stashed chocolate (left cupboard, third shelf, am I right?). That may give you an immediate sugar jolt, but you should choose something with a little more of a lasting effect. Go for a low-fat, low-protein, high-carbohydrate snack: Think toasted whole-wheat English muffin with a dollop of blueberry all-fruit preserves (or better, fresh blueberries). When high-carb foods aren't bogged down by protein or fat, they allow that amino acid called tryptophan (you know it from turkey) to flood into your brain, where it morphs into serotonin, a neurotransmitter that boosts mood and curbs food cravings. A bowl of air-popped popcorn is another good alternative.

When you're depressed: It's all about the fish. More and more evidence says that omega-3 fatty acids may help ease symptoms associated with depression. Omega-3s are found in fatty fish like salmon, herring, and tuna. One study, for example, showed that eating fish twice a week was associated with a lower risk of depression. If you're concerned about mercury (which is relatively high in fatty fish), stick to wild Pacific salmon, shrimp, summer flounder, farmed catfish, croaker, haddock, and mid-Atlantic blue crab, all of which contain omega-3s but are low in mercury.

When you're feeling dull: Here's the perfect place for your cup of joe (minus the whipped cream and flavors that sound like they belong in a bakery). Within a half hour of drinking a cup, your nervous system gets revved and you feel alert and better able to concentrate. How? The caffeine short-circuits a nerve chemical called adenosine that blocks your energy-boosting brain chemicals, helping you get a healthy rush. Just don't get into the cycle where you need coffee to pick you up, then feel a letdown, then reach for more coffee, and so on. To maintain a pleasant, temporary buzz, limit yourself to no more than three 5-ounce cups of coffee a day.

When you're sleepy: There's no doubt that a decrease in sleep equals an increase in irritability. To combat daytime fatigue, cut back on dinner. A big meal can keep you awake at night while your stomach churns on overload. Keep your dinner under 500 calories, and try to incorporate more foods containing the mineral copper. (Examples are chicken, bananas, and avocados.) There's some evidence that people who have a lower copper intake have a hard time getting to sleep and feel less rested when they wake up. Also add in a small low-fat, low-protein, high-carb evening snack (like a bit of sorbet or a small piece of fruit and graham crackers) to tap into serotonin's soothing effects.

When you're beyond tired: First off, if you're feeling too tired to even do your normal daily activities, you should see a doctor because fatigue can be a sign of a serious illness. It's one of the first signs of iron deficiency and anemia, the most common nutritional deficiency in the world, especially among women of childbearing age. The cause? Not getting enough iron from your food. As good as beans, grains, and vegetables are for you, the form of iron they provide is weak and hard to absorb. Animal protein not only contains more iron but also provides a special form that your body absorbs better than it does the iron from plants. If you're feeling listless, especially if you've cut back on meat, try eating shrimp, lean beef, dark chicken or turkey meat (without the skin), or fish. Adding a multivitamin with iron will also help. Another tactic: Try drinking more water. Chronic low fluid intake is a common but often overlooked cause of mild dehydration and fatigue.

Chapter 12

FITTING THE ABS DIET INTO EVERYDAY LIFE

How This Simple Eating Plan Makes Your Life Simpler, Too

IN PREVIOUS CHAPTERS, I OUTLINED WHY the Abs Diet works—and will work for you, for life. I gave an overview of the science and fed you some nifty terms like "glycemic index" and "basal metabolism." And I listed a whole eating plan complete with meals, snacks, and simple recipes.

But I also explained why most other diet plans are the nutritional equivalent of that tape recorder in *Mission: Impossible*—programmed to self-destruct in 5 seconds or 5 weeks or 5 years. Most diets just aren't designed to last over the long haul, or they're so complicated and restrictive that you'd have to quit your day job and disown half your friends in order to follow them to the letter. Many diets fail because they require us to work too hard and ignore the fact that we're already working too hard. What most of us feel, every day, is that our worlds are on the verge of spinning out of control. And what we want is to take back control—of our lives, our careers, our relationships, our bodies, our diets, ourselves.

One of the great side benefits of the Abs Diet is that it helps you reassert control over your life, which means taking control of your stress level. I can't emphasize strongly enough how important stress management is for your weight, your health, and the quality of life you'll lead.

ABS DIET SUCCESS STORY

"I'M ON THE ABS DIET FOR LIFE"

Name: Marian Nagel

Age: 44

Height: 5'6"

Starting weight: 148

6 weeks later: 136

As a mother of teenagers, Marian Nagel came to a point when she had to make a decision: "Do I want to be old and fat or old and healthy?"

So Nagel decided to get back in shape for herself—as well as to inspire her son to do so, too. After purchasing *Men's Health* to help him, Nagel learned about the Abs Diet, and they both tried it. She told her son, "This isn't a diet; it's a list of foods you need to eat more of." Within 6 weeks, Nagel's son dropped from 324 pounds to 292, and she dropped 12 pounds during the same time. (Since then, Nagel dropped down to 132, and she's now focused on losing just 4 more pounds.)

"Especially for women over 40, it gets harder and harder to lose that belly fat after having kids," says Nagel, who went from 27 percent body fat to about 20 during the initial part of the program and especially liked doing the interval training on a treadmill. "But I lost an incredible amount of inches. During the 6 weeks, I lost about 3½ inches off my waist. How nice it is to be curvy again. I see guys at the gym who can't do the abs work that I do."

Nagel also thinks the eating plan is perfect for women. "Women have a tendency to be nervous eaters more than men, and they assume they're going to eat more and take more calories if they eat six meals a day. But if you do it the proper way, you're nourishing your body, which speeds metabolism. You're eating to be sure your body is burning something all the time," Nagel says.

But for all the help the Abs Diet has given Nagel, she's especially happy for the way it's helped her son.

"The best thing for me is to set an example—not only to get myself in great shape but be a good example for him," Nagel says. "I absolutely love it, I'm still doing it; it's more of a lifestyle change than a temporary thing. I'm on the Abs Diet for life."

That's because our bodies simply aren't designed to handle the stress of modern life. See, when stress hits, one of the first things your body does is jack up its production of adrenaline. Adrenaline causes fat cells all over your body to squirt their stores of fatty acids into your bloodstream to be used as energy. This was great back when stress meant a charging saber-toothed tiger or an attacking horde of barbarians and your fight-or-flight mechanism switched on. But it's not so great in today's society, where the only tigers and barbarians you have to handle are the ones who sign your paycheck or spit milk across the table. You don't flee or fight; you just bear down to handle the situation. Meanwhile, your adrenal glands are producing yet another hormone to handle all that freshly released fat. It's called cortisol, but I want you to call it by its nickname: the belly-fat hormone.

In one Yale study, researchers asked 42 overweight people to perform an hour of stressful tasks—math problems, puzzles, and speech making. All the while, their cortisol levels were measured. The subjects who carried their extra weight in their bellies were discovered to be secreting more cortisol while under pressure. The theory runs like this: Stress hits, adrenaline mobilizes fat from all over the body, and cortisol takes the unused portion and stashes it with extreme prejudice toward the abdominal region. In a study of 438 firefighters, the ones who said

SNEAKY WAYS TO KEEP RESTAURANTS FROM SABOTAGING YOUR DIET

▶ Many chefs pour at least an ounce of butter (200 calories and 23 grams of fat) onto a steak just so the meat will look juicier. Ask in advance and tell the cook to lay off.

▶ Those harmless-looking shredded carrots that dress up your beef are probably deep-fried; ½ cup is 137 calories (four times that of raw carrots) and 12 grams of fat. Skip 'em.

▶ If you go to a restaurant that serves salads tossed with dressing, it's usually a much lighter coating than what most people end up dumping on themselves, even if you order it on the side.

they worried about their financial security gained 11.2 pounds over 7 years, compared with an average of 7.4 pounds gained by nonworriers. The key to managing your midsection, then, is managing your stress. Here are a few proven ways to keep your head—and your abs—when all around you are losing theirs.

Skip Letterman. A University of Chicago study published in the journal *Sleep* showed that people who slept only 4 hours had cortisol levels 37 percent higher than others who got a full 8 hours of shut-eye; those who stayed awake the whole night had levels 45 percent higher. Sleep specialists suggest that you strive for 8 hours per night.

Stop tossing and turning. How well you sleep matters, too. Another University of Chicago study showed that people who got plenty of deep sleep—the quality stuff without all the dreaming and rapid eye movement—secreted almost 65 percent more human growth hormone (HGH) than those who were short on good slumber. You want more HGH to help prevent the loss of muscle mass caused by cortisol.

Remember C, as in "crisis." If you're in a stressful time of life— wondering why the jury has been out so long, perhaps—load up on vitamin C. For managing stress, you probably top out the benefit with a daily intake of 1,000 milligrams, divided into small doses throughout the day.

Don't have that last drink. Booze dehydrates you. Your body thinks there's a water shortage emergency, which bumps up your cortisol. How much alcohol is too much? Most of the smart money says three drinks a day. Same dehydration idea applies to caffeine. For cortisol control, stick to 200 milligrams per day, about what you get in 2 cups of coffee.

Take the wheel. A sense of control over some of the stressors in your life helps. "If you blast a volunteer randomly with a noise, his stress hormones rise," says Robert Sapolsky, PhD, professor of biological and neurological sciences at Stanford University. "But if you give him a button and tell him that pressing it will decrease the likelihood of the noise, there's a smaller stress response to the same sound." Getting organized, even in small ways, may help you feel more like the captain of your ship.

Make a plan. "People manage stress more effectively if they can believe that things are improving," says Sapolsky. So make sure you always have something you're looking forward to. Hope makes stress manageable.

Get spiritual. Remember the simple wisdom of Simone Weil: Any undivided attention is prayer. If we can stop the tumble in our heads and every day briefly commit our complete attention to something—a 10-foot putt, a 10-penny nail, or a 10-year-old child—we may acquire the serenity many find in formal faith.

Chapter 18 will give you other great strategies for achieving peace of mind.

Chapter 13

TURBOCHARGING THE ABS DIET

How Exercise Can Strip Away Fat
and Add Lean Muscle

MAYBE THE LAST FEW months, years, or decades of your life have been one big snowstorm—a snowstorm of office parties and happy hours, of vending machine dinners, of finishing the cake and ice cream off your children's plates. When you're a kid, those storms can be fun, but as you get older, they're more of a mess than anything else. They dump pounds and pounds of fat onto your thighs, hips, and once-flat stomach, leaving your abdominal muscles buried deep under everything. No sun's going to melt your fat after a couple of days, and no snowblower's going to suck it up and shoot it over to the neighbor's lawn. (But how cool would that be?)

If you want to see the sidewalk, you have to shovel the snow. If you want to find your abs and flatten your belly, you have to burn the fat.

Eating right is critical, and yes, by following the nutrition principles of the Abs Diet and centering your meals around the Abs Diet Power-foods, you'll lose fat pretty effortlessly. But to maximize your weight loss and turn your fat into toned muscle, this book includes something other diet books ignore: a quick and easy exercise plan. Exercise will not only make you healthier; it'll also make you lose weight faster. It'll make you stronger. Most important, it'll make your body exchange your blobby fat for lean muscle—by converting energy that's stored in fat into energy that feeds muscle.

The Abs Diet Workout Principles

HAVING WORKED AT *Men's Health* for more than 10 years, I know all the latest trends in exercise, but I also scour the latest and most credible scientific research measuring the effectiveness of various workout plans. With that knowledge, I've constructed the exercise portion of the plan to help you burn fat at the highest levels possible in the least amount of time. I know you don't have time to spend hours a day exercising, so I want you to get the most out of every workout. And I know that flexibility and convenience are the keys to formulating a plan you can stick to, so I've created a workout you can do at your local gym—or in your living room. This plan allows you to keep your workouts short and focused, while still keeping you on target for your ultimate goal. Pound for pound, it's the best workout possible for finding your abs and flattening your stomach. These are the workout principles.

Focus on your diet first. The first 2 weeks of exercise are optional. If you already exercise regularly, you can jump right into the Abs Diet Workout, and you should, because you'll burn even more fat than with the Abs Diet alone. But if you're a beginner or you haven't exercised in

ABS FACTS

Stand tall: When you're walking, stand tall and picture a cape flowing off your shoulders, Superman-style, to ensure your best posture. A taller posture will give you the appearance of being slimmer, while also training your abs to stay taut and firm. Another good trick is to think of your back as a wall and your gut as a piece of furniture pushed up against the wall to keep it from buckling.

Watch your back: Contrary to popular belief, your abs aren't found just around your navel. They're an intricate system of muscles, connecting to your rib cage, your hips, and even your backbone. To have strong abs, you need not only belly exercises but also lower-back strength and exercises for your obliques (the abdominal muscles that run down the sides of your torso).

Tune in to muscle: Maybe you've heard of "muscle memory": the way your body learns to do a physical activity (like riding a bike) and never forgets.

a long time, take the first 2 weeks to adjust to your new eating plan before starting the workout. If you're champing at the bit to begin maximizing your weight loss, start getting in the exercise habit by walking briskly for up to 30 minutes a day.

Focus on muscles. I know a lot of people who have tried to lose weight by running, but many of them don't accomplish that even after following a good running program. They've either stayed at the same weight or gained some. I think that happens for a couple of reasons. For one, steady-state cardiovascular exercise doesn't burn fat the way strength training does. Your muscles are hungry little suckers, and in order to keep themselves well nourished, they want to churn and burn those calories you're ingesting. So adding some muscle means you'll burn more calories—at the gym, on the job, even in bed. This program focuses on working your large muscle groups—your legs, chest, back, and shoulders—because that's where you can build the most muscle in the least amount of time (without adding a lot of bulk). Plus, when you work your larger muscles, you fire up your metabolism by creating a longer calorie afterburn—one that can last right up to your very next workout!

Think about the small fraction of time you spend exercising. Even if

Well, your abs have a memory, too. If you consciously keep your abs firm throughout the day, they'll tend to stay firm even when you're relaxed.

Put exercise first: Research suggests that the best way to eat less at a meal is to work out right before it. This works in several ways: First, you're less hungry when your metabolism is revving, such as right after a workout. Second, you're thirstier, so you drink more water, which uses up space in your belly and relieves hunger. Third, with your metabolism revved, the calories you do eat get burned for energy pronto—not stored as fat.

Avoid the four-letter word: When you lose weight on a "diet," muscle is the first thing to go. It's more expensive for your body to retain than fat is, so when you run low on calories, your body dumps muscle mass and turns it into energy. When you go off the diet, you begin to gain back the pounds—but because you now have less calorie-burning muscle, the weight you gain is fat. By dieting, you've effectively turned muscle into fat.

you work out four or five times a week for an hour at a time, that's nothing compared to the amount of time you're not exercising every day. So in order to gain the most metabolic benefit, you want to maximize the calories you're burning when you're not working out.

Focus on spending less time in the gym. The Abs Diet Workout employs two simple concepts to maximize muscle growth and fat-burning and minimize the time you spend exercising.

Circuit training. This term refers to the practice of performing different exercises one right after another. For example, we'll have you do a set of leg exercises followed immediately by a set of an upper-body

---

ABS DIET SUCCESS STORY

"THE PROOF IS IN THE PANTS!"

Name: Jessica Guff

Age: 43

Height: 5'4"

Starting weight: 130

6 weeks later: 120

Jessica Guff doesn't believe in stepping on a scale. See, numbers don't give a total health picture, Guff says. What really matters is how you view yourself—not to mention how others view you, too. Take the time she was walking into a client's office. The people there hadn't seen her for a couple of weeks, and one employee said to another, "Who's that skinny woman over there?"

"It's Jessica," the other employee told her. "She's on this thing called the Abs Diet."

That exchange took place just 2 weeks after Guff started the Abs Diet—and she felt the effects immediately. Guff, 43, who runs marathons, has always been in good shape. But the effect of having two kids had taken a toll on her belly. "I was in pretty good shape, except for my stomach," she says. "But since going on the plan, I really noticed a difference. I could probably crunch walnuts with my abs."

The key for Guff was changing the way she approached eating. Sacrificing her own eating habits to get her kids out the door and keep up with her exercise, until you do 8 to 10 different exercises in a row. There are two reasons circuit training works. First, by keeping you moving and cutting down the rest periods between exercises, circuit training keeps your heart rate elevated throughout your training session, maximizing your fat burn while providing tremendous cardiovascular fitness benefits. Second, circuit training keeps your workout short; you won't waste time resting between sets of an exercise, which means you can get on with the rest of your busy life.

Compound exercises. Another key part of the strength-training program is compound exercises; that is, exercises that call into play

fitness training, she'd start the day with tea—and often little else. "I used to go out and run without eating anything, and that was really stupid," Guff says. "I was horrified to learn the truth—that exercising on an empty stomach causes you to burn muscle, not fat." But the simple strategies of the Abs Diet changed all that. "Now I'm having smoothies for breakfast, and it's made me fitter and stoked up my energy," Guff says.

Guff says she couldn't do a program in which she'd have to count calories or weigh food. "What I love about the Abs Diet is the flexibility," she says. "All I have to remember is the catchy acronym—ABS DIET POWER—and I can remember the 12 Powerfoods."

The results: Guff is leaner—and stronger. When her 56-pound daughter fell asleep on the couch, Guff was the one who picked her up and carried her to bed. "I thought, either I'm getting stronger or she's losing weight," she says.

And she's also more confident. "When women look at other women, they look at their boobs, their butts, and their waists—especially women who've had children. Every woman who's had a child cares about having a flat stomach."

But the true measure of her success came in the form of a pair of green satin cargo pants. Guff says, "They're kinda hot, but my stomach shows when I wear them. I have two kids, so I have no business flashing my midsection." But after 2 weeks on the plan, she decided to put them to the public test.

"All these people started complimenting me. A guy I went to college with said, 'Nice outfit.' My husband said I looked great," Guff says. "I'm going out tonight, and I'm wearing the pants again."

multiple muscle groups rather than just focusing on one. For example, with the Abs Diet Workout, we don't want you to exercise your chest, and then your shoulders, and then your triceps, and then your forearms. We want you to hit many different muscles at the same time and then get out of the gym. What's best is that workouts that build 2 to 3 pounds of lean muscle for women take only 20 minutes three times a week. Not only do compound exercises make your workout more fun and more challenging, they will also increase the demands on your muscles—even though you're not actually doing more work. (For instance, the squat hits a whopping 256 muscles with just one movement!) Greater muscle demand triggers your body to produce more human growth hormone—a potent fat burner.

If the only weight you've ever picked up comes from lemon meringue pie and not in the gym, don't worry that you're not familiar with working with weights. You can start by lifting any amount of weight that you're comfortable with—whether it's a pair of light dumbbells or a couple of cans of beans (Powerfood!). Even if you start small, you'll grow stronger, start to build lean muscle, and keep your metabolism revved. As you progress, you'll build and burn more.

Focus on intensity. Time and time again, research has shown that higher-intensity workouts promote weight loss better than steady-state activities. In a Canadian study from Laval University, researchers measured differences in fat loss between two groups of exercisers following two different workout programs. The first group rode stationary bikes four or five times a week and burned 300 to 400 calories per 30- to 45-minute session. The second group did the same, but only one or two times a week, and they filled the rest of their sessions with short intervals of high-intensity cycling. They hopped on their stationary bikes and pedaled as quickly as they could for 30 to 90 seconds, rested, and then repeated the process several times per exercise session. As a result, they burned 225 to 250 calories while cycling, but they had burned more fat at the end of the study than the workers in the first group. In fact, even though they exercised less, their fat loss was nine times greater. Researchers said that the majority of the fat burning took place after the workout.

The Abs Diet Workout recommends that you add one simple interval workout per week to complement your strength training. These are workouts of traditional cardiovascular exercise (running, swimming, biking) in which you alternate between periods of high intensity and periods of rest. (I'll explain more about how to create an effective interval workout in the next chapter.)

If You Don't Already Exercise

THE BEST PART about the 6-week Abs Diet Workout is that, for the first 2 weeks at least, you don't actually have to exercise. If you're not doing anything right now, it's not critical that you start immediately. Instead, I want you to concentrate on acclimating your body and your schedule to the Abs Diet.

On the other hand, why wait to fire up your fat-burning mechanisms? If you want to start a light strength-training program, do this workout three times a week: Alternate between three sets of Pushups (on your knees if you're unable to do them with straight legs at first) and three sets of Squats with no weight. Both exercises use your body weight as resistance and will get your body accustomed to a strength-training program. Do 8 to 10 repetitions of Pushups, followed by 15 to 20 repetitions of Squats. When that becomes too easy, increase the repetitions of Pushups, and hold on to some form of weight—light dumbbells are best—while doing Squats. This light workout, especially in combination with 30 minutes of brisk walking, will really fire up your fat burners.

If You're Already in the Exercise Habit

MAYBE YOU LIFT weights once or twice a week. Maybe you jog a few miles every morning. Maybe you're favored to win the gold in the decathlon this summer. I dunno. What I do know is that no matter what your workout is now, you're probably going to build more muscle and burn more fat if you switch to the Abs Diet Workout.

Even if your current exercise program has been working well for you, experts agree that mixing up your workout every month or so is the best way to maximize your results. That's because gains in strength and overall fitness come from challenging your body to perform in ways it's not used to. Performing the same workout over and over again doesn't train your body to reach its potential; it just trains your body to be really, really good at performing that one workout. So I want you to consider switching your current workout over to the Abs Diet Workout, at least for a few weeks. I guarantee the results you'll see will be astounding.

The Abs Diet Workout: Suggested Weekly Schedule

YOU CAN MIX and match the different workouts to meet your lifestyle needs. When you construct your schedule, make sure to:

▶ Leave at least 48 hours between weight workouts of the same body parts. Your muscles need time to recover and repair themselves after a workout.

▶ Take 1 day each week to rest with no formal exercise.

▶ Warm up for 5 minutes before starting to exercise, either through a light jog, riding on a stationary bike, jumping rope, or doing slow jumping jacks.

The three components of your weekly schedule include:

1. Strength training: three times a week. These are total-body workouts with one workout that puts extra emphasis on your legs.

2. Additional cardiovascular exercise: optional, on non-strength-training days. Examples are cycling, running, swimming, walking, and using cardio machines. An interval workout is recommended for 1 day a week, and light cardiovascular exercise like walking is recommended for 2 of your 3 off days.

3. Abs exercises: twice a week. I recommend doing them before your strength training or interval workouts (more on abs exercises in Chapter 15).

THE ABS DIET WORKOUT

The Easiest, Most Effective Workout Plan Ever

YOU SEE EVERY KIND OF PERSON IN the gym. The people with no fat. The people with no necks. The people with lots of fat. The people with lots of necks. And it seems they all get there a different way. I know that gym-goers have as many different workout philosophies as FOX has reality TV shows, but the one person I really know I can help is the overweight person who's working on tiny muscles in the corner. Working very small muscle groups—say, the one in your forearms or calves—is like putting on makeup before you take a shower. There's no point working on the fine points until you've taken care of the bigger issues.

That's why I've built a total-body strength training workout: to increase your lean muscle mass as efficiently as possible. It's simple: To show off your abs and flatten your belly, you have to burn fat. To burn fat, you have to build some muscle. Remember that adding just 1 pound of muscle will force your body to burn up to an additional 50 calories a day, every day.

This workout emphasizes the larger muscle groups of your body—chest, back, and legs. In one workout during the week, you'll give extra attention to your legs. I know what you're thinking: My abs are up here. Why do I care about working what's down there? Because most of your body's muscle is found below your belly button. Your lower body is where you'll build the most muscle in the least amount of time; working this giant muscle mass triggers the release of hormones that stimulate muscle growth throughout your body, kick your fat burners into overdrive, and give you that thin-as-a-dime stomach you want—in no time flat. Indeed, leg exercises are the key to total-body strength: In one Norwegian study, people who focused on lower-body work gained more upper-body strength than did those who emphasized upper-body exercises in their workouts. That doesn't mean you'll ignore your upper body entirely, though. With the upper-body workout, you'll also work your largest muscles—your chest, back, and shoulders—to burn more fat. If you follow this program, you'll still notice more growth and definition in your whole body—even your arms, even your shoulders, and yes, even your abs—and you'll begin to reshape your body.

Here, you're going to do circuit training to optimize your muscle-building potential. That is, you'll perform one set of an exercise and then move immediately to the next exercise, with just 30 seconds of rest. Follow the order of the exercises I've listed on the following pages; that will allow you to work different body parts from set to set. (A complete

THE LITERALLY LAST-MINUTE WEIGHT-LOSS PLAN

Whether on the red carpet or at a photo shoot, models and actresses are used to showing lots of skin. Often, they'll use these last few tricks to make their bodies look their best. Here are instant ways to enhance and hone your appearance for the big day—whether it's at the beach or in a wedding gown.

Pump fast. Do quick strength moves like pushups or squats right before you show off. Increase your speed and reps in order to force blood into your muscles. More blood equals more tone.

Drink water. Guzzling a few glasses of H_2O before hitting the beach will help flush your system and relieve bloating.

Know your bloat foods. Avoid beans, for example, if they're hard for you to digest or if they make you bloat. Dairy has the same effect for some. And minimize your sodium intake. While there's no Recommended Dietary Allowance, most nutritionists suggest you stay under 2,500 or 3,000 mg to avoid bloating (most of us have 5,000 milligrams a day).

set of exercise descriptions and instructional photos begins on page 186.) By alternating between body parts, you'll keep your body in constant work mode and be able to perform the movements back-to-back without rest. Here's why circuit training works so well: You'll save time because you'll cut the amount of rest you need when you alternate muscle groups. More important, you'll keep your heart rate elevated throughout the workout, so you'll burn even more fat while you're exercising—whether you're in the gym or in your own living room.

In the first 2 weeks of the program, do the circuit twice. Move from exercise to exercise with no more than 30 seconds of rest in between. When you complete one circuit, rest for 1 to 2 minutes, then complete the second circuit. After the first 2 weeks, when you've become comfortable doing two complete circuits during a workout, increase your workload to three circuits per workout. In every exercise, use a weight that you can handle comfortably for the number of repetitions noted. When that becomes too easy, increase the weight on each set by 10 percent or less. Here's a sample schedule of how you might arrange your workouts.

MONDAY:
Total-Body Strength Training Workout with Ab Emphasis
Complete one set of each ab exercise*, then complete the rest of the circuit twice.

EXERCISE	REPETITIONS	REST	SETS
Traditional Crunch*	12–15	none	1
Bent-Leg Knee Raise*	12–15	none	1
Oblique V-Up*	10 each side	none	1
Bridge*	1 or 2	none	1
Back Extension*	12–15	none	1
Squat	10–12	30 seconds	2
Bench Press	10	30 seconds	2
Pulldown	10	30 seconds	2
Military Press	10	30 seconds	2

(continued)

EXERCISE	REPETITIONS	REST	SETS
Upright Row	10	30 seconds	2
Triceps Pushdown	10–12	30 seconds	2
Leg Extension	10–12	30 seconds	2
Biceps Curl	10	30 seconds	2
Leg Curl	10–12	30 seconds	2

TUESDAY (OPTIONAL):
Light Cardiovascular Exercise Such as Walking
Try for 30 minutes at a brisk pace.

WEDNESDAY:
Total-Body Strength Training Workout with Ab Emphasis
Complete one set of each ab exercise*, then complete the
rest of the circuit twice.

EXERCISE	REPETITIONS	REST	SETS
Standing Crunch*	12–15	none	1
Pulse-Up*	12	none	1
Saxon Side Bend*	6–10 each side	none	1
Side Bridge*	1 or 2 each side	none	1
Back Extension*	12–15	none	1
Squat	10–12	30 seconds	2
Bench Press	10	30 seconds	2
Pulldown	10	30 seconds	2
Military Press	10	30 seconds	2
Upright Row	10	30 seconds	2
Triceps Pushdown	10–12	30 seconds	2
Leg Extension	10–12	30 seconds	2
Biceps Curl	10	30 seconds	2
Leg Curl	10–12	30 seconds	2

THURSDAY (OPTIONAL):
Light Cardiovascular Exercise Such as Walking
Try for 30—45 minutes at a brisk pace.

FRIDAY:
Total-Body Strength Training Workout with Leg Emphasis
Repeat entire circuit twice.

EXERCISE	REPETITIONS	REST	SETS
Squat	10–12	30 seconds	2
Bench Press	10	30 seconds	2
Pulldown	10	30 seconds	2
Traveling Lunge	10–12 each leg	30 seconds	2
Military Press	10	30 seconds	2
Upright Row	10	30 seconds	2
Step-Up	10–12 each leg	30 seconds	2
Triceps Pushdown	10–12	30 seconds	2
Leg Extension	10–12	30 seconds	2
Biceps Curl	10	30 seconds	2
Leg Curl	10–12	30 seconds	2

SATURDAY (OPTIONAL):
Abs Workout Plus Interval Workout
Complete one set of each ab exercise, then choose one
interval workout from the selection on pages 209 and 210.

EXERCISE	REPETITIONS	REST	SETS
Traditional Crunch	12–15	none	1
Bent-Leg Knee Raise	12	none	1
Oblique V-Up	6–10 each side	none	1
Bridge	1 or 2	none	1
Back Extension	12–15	none	1

SUNDAY: OFF

Basic Exercises

SQUAT

Hold a barbell with an overhand grip so that it rests comfortably on your upper back. Set your feet shoulder-width apart, and keep your knees slightly bent, back straight, and eyes focused straight ahead. Slowly lower your body as if you were sitting back into a chair, keeping your back in its natural alignment and your lower legs nearly perpendicular to the floor. When your thighs are parallel to the floor, pause, then return to the starting position.

*HOME VARIATION: Same, but with one
dumbbell in each hand, your palms
facing your outer thighs.*

BENCH PRESS

Lie on your back on a flat bench with your feet on the floor. Grab the barbell with an overhand grip, your hands just beyond shoulder-width apart. Lift the bar off the uprights and hold it at arm's length over your chest. Slowly lower the bar to your chest. Pause, then push the bar back to the starting position.

HOME VARIATION: Just do standard Pushups: Get in a Pushup position with your hands about shoulder-width apart. Bend at the elbows while keeping your back straight, until your chin almost touches the floor, then push back up.

PULLDOWN

Stand facing a lat pulldown machine. Reach up and grasp the bar with an overhand grip that's 4 to 6 inches wider than your shoulders. Sit on the seat, letting the resistance of the bar extend your arms above your head. When you're in position, pull the bar down until it touches your upper chest. Hold this position for a second, then return to the starting position.

HOME VARIATION: Bent-Over Row. Stand with your knees slightly bent and shoulder-width apart. Bend over so that your back is almost parallel to the floor. Holding a dumbbell in each hand, let your arms hang toward the floor. With your palms facing in, pull the dumbbells toward you until they touch the outside of your chest. Pause, then return to the starting position.

MILITARY PRESS

Sitting on an exercise bench, hold a barbell at shoulder height with your hands shoulder-width apart. Press the weight straight overhead so that your arms are almost fully extended, hold for a count of one, then bring it down to the front of your shoulders.

HOME VARIATION: Sitting on a sturdy chair instead of a bench, hold one dumbbell in each hand, about level with your ears. Push the dumbbells straight overhead so that your arms are almost fully extended, hold for a count of one, then return to the starting position.

UPRIGHT ROW

Grab a barbell with an overhand grip, and stand with your feet shoulder-width apart and your knees slightly bent. Let the barbell hang at arm's length on top of your thighs, thumbs pointed toward each other. Bending your elbows, lift your upper arms straight out to the sides, and pull the barbell straight up until your upper arms are parallel to the floor and the bar is just below chin level. Pause, then return to the starting position.

HOME VARIATION: Same, using one dumbbell in each hand.

TRICEPS PUSHDOWN

While standing, grip a bar attached to a high pulley cable or lat machine with your hands about 6 inches apart. With your elbows tucked against your sides, bring the bar down until it is directly in front of you. With your forearms parallel to the floor (the starting position), push the bar down until your arms are extended straight down with the bar near your thighs. Don't lock your elbows. Return to the starting position.

HOME VARIATION: *Triceps Kickback.* Stand with your knees slightly bent and shoulder-width apart. Bend over so that your back is almost parallel to the floor. Bend your elbows to about 90-degree angles, raising them to just above the level of your back. This is the starting position. Extend your forearms backward, keeping your upper arms stationary. When they're fully extended, your arms should be parallel to the ground. Pause, then return to the starting position.

LEG EXTENSION

Sitting on a leg extension machine with your feet under the footpads, lean back slightly, and lift the pads with your feet until your legs are extended. Return to the starting position.

HOME VARIATION: Wall Squat. Stand with your back flat against a wall. Squat down so that your thighs are parallel to the ground. Hold that position for as long as you can. That's one set. Aim for 20 seconds to start and work your way up to 45 seconds. Return to the starting position.

BICEPS CURL

Stand while holding a barbell in front of you, palms facing out, with your hands shoulder-width apart and your arms hanging in front of you. Curl the weight toward your shoulders, hold for a second, then return to the starting position.

HOME VARIATION: Same, only use a set of dumbbells instead.

LEG CURL

Lie facedown on a leg curl machine and hook your ankles under the padded bar. Keeping your stomach and pelvis against the bench, slowly raise your feet toward your butt, curling up the weight. Come up so that your feet nearly touch your butt and slowly return to the starting position.

HOME VARIATION: Lie down with your stomach on the floor. Put a light dumbbell between your feet (so that the top end of the dumbbell rests on the bottom of your feet). Squeeze your feet together and curl them up toward your butt. Slowly return to the starting position.

TRAVELING LUNGE

Rest a barbell across your upper back. Stand, with your feet hip-width apart, at one end of the room; you need room to walk about 20 steps. Step forward with your left foot and lower your body so that your left thigh is parallel to the floor and your right thigh is perpendicular to the floor (your right knee should bend and almost touch the floor). Stand and bring your right foot up next to your left, then repeat with the right leg lunging forward.

HOME VARIATION: Use dumbbells, holding one in each hand with your arms at your sides. If you don't have enough space, do the move in one place, alternating your lead foot with each lunge.

STEP-UP

Use a step or bench that's 18 inches off the ground. Place your left foot on the step so that your knee is bent at 90 degrees. Your knee should not advance past the toes of your left foot. Push off with your left foot and bring your right foot onto the step, keeping your back straight. Now step down with the left foot, followed by the right. Alternate the leading foot, or do all of the repetitions leading with one foot and then alternating. Once you're comfortable, add dumbbells.

HOME VARIATION: Same, only use a staircase instead of a step (if you don't have one).

The Interval Workout

THEY SAY THAT slow and steady wins the race. But the cardiovascular key to fat burning is using interval workouts—workouts that alternate high-intensity levels with lower-intensity effort. As I mentioned earlier, that formula keeps your body burning calories long after you've stopped working out. Interval workouts mimic sports-start-and-stop motions with periods of sprinting or close-to-sprinting speeds followed by light jogging or rest. You can use interval workouts any way you want—running, cycling, swimming, on elliptical trainers, even walking if you alternate a speed walk and slow walk. You can also vary the intensity levels in different combinations. To start, here are three options for setting your workout. (If you use exercise machines, don't choose the interval workout; choose the manual one and create your own intensities by adjusting it yourself. It'll give you greater control over the speeds and will help you burn fat faster.) You'll derive benefits in as little as a 20-minute interval workout. As you build up endurance and strength, you can add time to your workout.

ABS DIET SUCCESS STORY

"THE JELLY DOUGHNUT AROUND MY BELLY BUTTON FADED AWAY"

Name: Jamie Bellavance

Age: 22

Height: 5'5"

Weight, Week 1: 150

Weight, Week 6: 143

Body fat percentage, Week 1: 29 percent

Body fat percentage, Week 2: 24 percent

During her freshman year at Syracuse University in New York, Jamie Bellavance was petrified of the freshman 15. So she worked out every day and had salads for meals—while her friends would take 2-hour naps and hover around the fried chicken station at dinner. And she lost weight during her freshman year.

Interval Variation I: Standard

The following is a typical interval workout. You alternate the same period of low intensity with the same period of higher intensity.

3–5 minutes warmup (light jog, low intensity, gradually increasing at the end of the warmup period)

1 minute moderate or high intensity followed by 1 minute low intensity (repeat 6–8 times)

3–5 minutes cooldown (light jog, low intensity, gradually decreasing by the end of the cooldown period)

Interval Variation II: Pyramid

This pyramid structure allows you to start with short bursts of speed, and then you'll peak at the longest surge of energy in the middle of your workout before coming back down.

3–5 minutes warmup

30 seconds high intensity

"Little by little, I became a little less strict on myself. I figured I only lived once—and headed out to party 4 nights a week," she says. "We'd have our own pitchers at happy hour, and polish the night off with a few slices of pizza."

By the end of her senior year, Bellavance had gained 10 pounds. After graduation, she thought she'd lose weight because she was removing the temptations of college life, but the weight never disappeared.

An internship at *Men's Health* persuaded her to try the Abs Diet. "I was skeptical at first because I had been working out all summer with no results," she says.

But within 2 weeks of lifting weight, she started losing weight. And she found the interval training to be more fun than steady runs. "Smoothies? Dear god, I couldn't wait until the next morning so I could drink one. Tastes like ice cream for breakfast," she says.

By the 4th week, her face had thinned out, and she proudly whipped out her bikini for a Key West trip.

She says, "My entire body took on a more toned physique as the jelly doughnut around my belly button faded away."

1 minute low intensity

45 seconds high intensity

1 minute low intensity

60 seconds high intensity

1 minute low intensity

90 seconds high intensity

1 minute low intensity

60 seconds high intensity

1 minute low intensity

45 seconds high intensity

1 minute low intensity

30 seconds high intensity

3–5 minutes cooldown

Interval Variation III: Faster, Harder

Sports are unpredictable. This interval simulates some of that unpredictability by having you do different times and different intensities. You can mix and match the order and repetitions as much as you want. Rest longer after the periods in which you use the most energy.

3–5 minutes warmup

2 minutes moderate or high intensity followed by 2 minutes low intensity (repeat once)

30 seconds high intensity followed by 30 seconds low intensity (repeat four times)

60-yard sprints (or 10 seconds if not running) followed by 90 seconds rest (repeat 6–10 times)

3–5 minutes cooldown

What Kind of a Woman Are You?

You can make some adjustments to the Abs Diet exercises and circuit, depending on what body type you are.

If your body type is lean and narrow: You want to build strength and curves with slow weight training. By lifting weight slowly, you'll challenge muscle fibers and help build them up faster—not to mention gaining some super muscle definition. Do the Abs Diet Circuit, but try doing each exercise with a slow, controlled movement. Try doing each repetition by taking 3 seconds to raise the weight and 3 seconds to lower it.

If your body type is classically curvy: You want to balance and tone by burning fat and calories with a fast-paced routine. A quick cardio kickboxing interval like the one starting on page 213 burns fat and calories. Pump up the music and run through these exercises one after the other. Do two or three circuits.

If your body type is athletic: You want to get lean and energized with the active yoga, dance, and Pilates postures beginning on page 218, to maintain and tone your athletic build.

DUMBBELL SMARTS

When it comes to versatility, ease of use, and pure effectiveness, no muscle-building equipment beats dumbbells. On a practical level, they're inexpensive, virtually indestructible, and compact. (Just try stuffing a Soloflex under the bed!) Here are eight reasons why smart folks surround themselves with dumbbells.

1. Dumbbells give you a more complete workout. You may think of dumbbells only in terms of biceps curls, but they're effective for working your legs (Lunges, Calf Raises), back (Deadlifts), and abdominals (Side Bends, Weighted Crunches) as well.

2. Dumbbells challenge your muscles more. One of the biggest challenges to weight lifters is a phenomenon called plateauing. When your body becomes used to a given workout, it stops being challenged, and your muscles stop growing. Because there are hundreds of different exercises you can do with dumbbells, you can keep changing and updating your workout, so your muscles stay challenged—and keep growing. For example, there are 15 or 20 variations of biceps curls you can do with dumbbells, as opposed to only a handful you can do with a barbell and only one or two at most on an exercise machine.

3. Dumbbells build greater strength. Because they allow for a greater range of motion during exercise, dumbbells challenge your muscles in ways no other equipment can. For example, a barbell becomes restricting during a bench press because you can bring the weight down only so far before your chest gets in the way. But when you're holding a dumbbell in each

(continued)

DUMBBELL SMARTS *(CONT.)*

hand, you can bring the weight down lower during each repetition, calling into play more muscle fiber and stimulating more growth.

4. Dumbbells build strength faster. Negative resistance training refers to the stress you put on your muscles during the lowering, or negative, phase of an exercise. And negative resistance may grow muscle even more effectively than the positive, or lifting, phase of an exercise. With dumbbells, you can add extra negative resistance into your workout. Let's say you've done 10 biceps curls with your left hand, and you can't possibly lift the weight one more time. You can now cheat, using your right hand to help your left lift the weight one more time, and simply lower the dumbbell using your left hand only. Doing so will help you squeeze out that last little bit of benefit from your workout.

5. Dumbbells can give you a healthier heart. Plenty of studies have shown that weight training reduces blood pressure and indirectly strengthens the heart. Researchers have also shown that a dumbbell workout can yield additional benefits, including a lower lipid profile (less gum for your arteries) and increased oxygen uptake. Dumbbells do a better job at this than other weight training, again because of the greater range of motion they allow.

6. Dumbbells make you smarter. Your muscles, anyway. Dumbbells make you work in three dimensions: They don't lock you into the up-and-down or side-to-side motions that exercise machines do. That means your muscles learn to function well in real life, whether you're catching the winning pass in the neighborhood game or catching the kids before they fall off the swings.

7. Dumbbells keep your body in balance. By forcing each arm to lift its fair share, dumbbells help to immediately identify strength imbalances that may have developed from sports, from simple acts like driving or carrying a briefcase, or from lifting with barbells or machines. When pressing a barbell overhead, for example, you can compensate for a weaker left arm by pushing more with your right side—and just make the imbalance worse. When you're pressing two dumbbells overhead, however, each side of your body has to work independently—and each side gets the same amount of exercise.

8. Dumbbells help prevent injury. Exercise machines are calibrated to target one muscle exclusively, to maximize growth. On a practical level, it's important to also strengthen the small muscles, ligaments, and tendons. Machines may miss these, setting you up for injury. Dumbbells strengthen you everywhere, protecting you from harm.

Cardio Kickboxing Interval for Curvy Women

DUCK

Stand with your legs shoulder-width apart, elbows to your sides, and fists clenched just below the chin, in a classic kickboxing guard stance. Squat back into your hips, down, and then up. Do eight reps.

BOB AND WEAVE

While keeping your elbows stationary against your sides and fists anchored below the chin, slide the right leg out and bring the left in, tapping it alongside the right. Repeat, alternating sides, 10 times.

JACK SQUAT

With your elbows against your sides and fists anchored below the chin, spread your feet out while bending your knees and keeping your weight on the balls of your feet. Bounce twice with feet spread apart, then bring your feet back together, bouncing twice again. Repeat complete jacks, out and in, 10 times.

KNEE STRIKE

With elbows against your sides and fists anchored just below the chin, slightly bend the left leg, balancing your weight on it. Bring the right leg up and lift the knee up toward the ceiling, then return the leg onto the ball of the foot behind you. Repeat sides. Do this four times.

SCISSOR JACK

Raise your arms above your head toward the ceiling, and step the left foot in front of the right, keeping your knees soft. Hop up and switch legs, shifting your weight with each switch. Do this 10 times.

Active Postures for Athletic Women

WARRIOR I LUNGE

Begin with one foot forward so that your forward thigh is parallel to the ground. Turn your back heel down and square your hips to the front. Open up your chest by raising your arms over your head and putting your palms together. Lean your head back and lengthen your lower back by moving your tailbone toward the ground (keep your back leg straight). Inhale as you push and straighten the left leg up away from the floor, then exhale as you bend forward again. Do this four times, then switch and repeat, using opposite legs.

WARRIOR II

Begin with your left foot forward, knee bent (not beyond the toes), and right leg straightened behind you, with the right foot almost reaching the back edge of the mat, toes turned outward. Square your shoulders and hips, pivoting your body to the right. Fully extend both arms (left in front of you, right behind you), keeping them parallel above the floor. Inhale as you push your left leg up away from the floor, and exhale as you bend the knee back down, keeping your arms level with your shoulders. Do this four times, then switch and repeat, using opposite legs.

ATHLETIC PLIÉ

With your toes turned outward at 10 and 2 o'clock on your mat (legs spread horizontally, almost reaching each end of the mat), lift your arms above your head to begin, with palms facing away from you. Keeping your feet firmly planted, bend both knees outward and bring your arms down, exhaling as you do so. Stop your arms when elbows align with shoulders. Bend both knees, hold, and return to your original position 8 to 10 times.

Chapter **15**

TARGETING YOUR ABS
A 50-"6-Pack" of Exercises

HEN I WAS IN COLLEGE, I had a friend who argued that he knew the key to a six-pack: "All you have to do is 1,000 crunches a day for a month." He said it in a way that made you believe him—that if only you were disciplined enough to put in the time every day to concentrate on your abdominal muscles, then you'd eventually chisel away a gut of stone. His theory was that it all boiled down to volume and discipline. He went on to say that the iconic ab exercise would do more than just build abs—that it was also the fix-all to weight problems, that you could simply crunch away years of bingeing on pizza, fries, and ranch dressing by the gallon.

In a lot of ways (a heck of a lot of ways, actually), my friend was wrong. For one, crunching won't burn fat. And you won't develop abs by doing the same exercise over and over—let alone the same exercise every day. And 1,000 repetitions? C'mon. There's only one thing many of us would do 1,000 times a day if it were physically possible, and it wouldn't be a crunch. But he was right in one sense: If you want abs that will make you stronger, healthier, and better looking, you do have to work them. And that does take discipline—but not as much as you'd think.

Though your midsection works as one unified core, it does help to think of your abdominal center in regions. To build a defined belly, you need to work the entire region. The three visible regions consist of the upper abs, lower abs, and obliques (the muscles along the side of your torso). But there are also a number of supporting muscles that, when developed, will add strength to your abdominals: your lower back and the transverse abdominis—muscles that run underneath your abdomen horizontally to give support to your entire midsection.

You already have all of these muscles; you just need them to come front and center. That's why your priorities have to revolve around the first two components: the nutrition principles and the fat-burning workout. Once you strip away the fat, your abs can grow and show. Unlike what my friend said, you won't get a six-pack by working your abdominal muscles every day. Instead, follow these guidelines for adding the final component.

REACQUAINT YOURSELF WITH YOUR ABS

Your abdominal muscles are a lot like a skilled group of employees. The harder they work, the better they make you look, and vice versa.

This is because you use your abs in virtually every movement that matters. Lifting. Running. Jumping. Reproducing. (It takes a lot of midsection stability to stand over that copy machine. Especially when it's printing on both sides of the page.) So the stronger they are, the harder and longer you'll be able to play. Here's a quick course in the anatomy of your abs.

Rectus abdominis. This is the six-pack muscle that helps your upper body bend (like in a crunch) and also helps keep good posture. It's what people think of when they think of abs.

External obliques. These muscles start on the ribs and extend diagonally down the sides of your waist. If a movement happens at your waist, the external obliques are involved. The torso rotation that's key to golf, tennis, and hockey is mostly a function of the external obliques. Even the basic crunching motion, attributed to the rectus abdominis (the six-pack muscle), wouldn't be possible without a strong contraction of the external obliques to stabilize the torso.

Internal obliques. These lie between the rib cage and the external obliques and also extend diagonally down the sides of your waist. Similar to the externals, the internal obliques are involved in torso rotation. You use these muscles when you breathe deeply.

Transverse abdominis. It's a thin muscle that runs horizontally, surrounding your abdomen. It's also known as the girdle because it functions as a compressor for the abdomen, keeping everything in place.

Work your abs 2 or 3 days a week. Abs are like any other muscle in your body. They'll grow when they're at rest, not when you're working them. So working them every day doesn't give them a chance to grow and get strong. You will develop abs by working them two or three times a week. I'd recommend adding the ab circuit to the beginning of your workout. Saving them until the end of the workout means there's more possibility that you'll skimp and take shortcuts.

Hit the whole region. You have five regions of your abdominals that you're going to work. For each workout, pick one exercise per region to ensure that you're hitting every area.

Pick different exercises every workout. We're giving you 56 different exercises for your abdominals, but you need to pick only 5 exercises each workout. The key is variety: Changing your routine doesn't allow your abs to get comfortable, so they'll continue to grow after each workout.

Do a circuit. In the first week of workouts, just do one set of each exercise (10 to 15 repetitions, depending on the exercise). In the second and third weeks, do two sets if you'd like, but perform them in a circuit so that you're doing each exercise once before repeating an exercise. After that, you can do three circuits. Even then, your ab workouts shouldn't take more than 5 minutes.

Go slow. Each rep of an ab exercise should last slightly longer than Kajagoogoo lasted on the radio—4 to 6 seconds. Any faster, and you run the risk of letting momentum do the work. The slower you go, the higher the intensity. The higher the intensity, the stronger the stomach.

In this chapter you'll find 56 exercises—a 50-"6-pack" of exercises—so that you'll never get bored and so that you'll work your abdominals as efficiently as possible. Remember that this portion of the workout is what will make your belly as tight as a size-too-small pair of high heels. Think of the ab exercise portion of the plan as the toy at the bottom of the cereal box, the paycheck at the end of the week, the finish line at the end of the marathon. It's the motivation. It's the reward. It's the goal that no scale could ever show.

How to Do the Workout

PICK ONE EXERCISE from each group of the listings below and do the exercise for the specified number of repetitions. Do one set of each exercise, and then repeat the circuit.

Note: Many of these exercises target different regions of the abdominals during the same movement, but they're grouped based on what areas they primarily target. They've also been grouped by levels of difficulty so that you can change your workouts as you get stronger. For each exercise, pause at the end of the movement and return to the starting position. That counts as one repetition, unless otherwise noted.

The Abs Circuit

Upper Abs (pages 225 to 234)

Lower Abs (pages 235 to 244)

Obliques (pages 245 to 250)

Transverse Abdominis (pages 251 to 258)

Lower Back (pages 259 to 262)

Upper Abs

TRADITIONAL CRUNCH

Lie on your back with your knees bent and your hands behind your ears. Slowly crunch up, bringing your shoulder blades off the ground.

12–15 repetitions [*Beginner*]

STANDING CRUNCH

Attach a rope handle to a high cable pulley. Stand with your back to the weight stack and hold the ends of the rope behind your head. Crunch down.

12–15 repetitions [*Beginner*]

MODIFIED RAISED-FEET CRUNCHES

Lie on your back with your knees bent and your hands behind your ears. Raise your feet just a few inches off the floor and hold them there. Crunch up, then lower your torso back to the floor, keeping your feet raised throughout the movement.

12–15 repetitions [*Beginner to intermediate*]

DECLINE CRUNCH

Lie on your back on a decline board, with your ankles locked under the padded support bars and your fingertips cupped behind your ears. Lift your shoulder blades off the bench, keeping your lower body flat. Don't jerk your body to build momentum. Hold the contraction for a second.

12–15 repetitions [*Beginner to intermediate*]

LYING CABLE CRUNCH

Attach a rope handle to the low pulley. Lie on the floor with your head near the low pulley, your knees bent, and your feet flat on the floor. Hold the handle over your chest so that the point of the rope attachment is at the base of your neck. Crunch your rib cage toward your pelvis, lifting your shoulder blades a few inches off the floor.

12–15 repetitions [*Intermediate to advanced*]

WEIGHTED CRUNCH

Lie on your back with your knees bent, holding a weight plate or dumbbell across your chest. Slowly crunch up, bringing your shoulder blades off the ground. Use progressively heavier weight.

12–15 repetitions [*Intermediate to advanced*]

LONG-ARM WEIGHTED CRUNCH

Lie on your back with your knees bent. Hold a light dumbbell in each hand and stretch your arms straight back behind you. Crunch your rib cage toward your pelvis. Don't generate momentum with your arms.

12–15 repetitions [*Intermediate to advanced*]

TOE TOUCH

Lie on your back with your legs raised directly over your hips; your knees should be slightly bent. Raise your arms straight up, pointing toward your toes, and relax your head and neck. Use your upper abs to raise your rib cage toward your pelvis, lift your shoulder blades off the floor, and reach toward your toes. Hold for a second. Lower your shoulders to the floor and repeat.

12–15 repetitions [*Intermediate to advanced*]

MEDICINE BALL BLAST

Set an adjustable ab bench at a 45-degree angle. Lie down on it with your head toward the floor and hook your feet under the padded support bars. Hold a medicine ball at your chest as you lower yourself. As you come up, chest-pass the ball straight up over your head. Catch it at the top of the movement, then lower yourself and repeat.

12–15 repetitions [*Advanced*]

SICILIAN CRUNCH

Slide your feet under the handles of heavy dumbbells. Place a rolled-up towel under your lower back and hold a dumbbell across your chest. Raise your upper body as high as possible by crunching your rib cage toward your pelvis. At the top of the move, straighten your arms and raise the dumbbell above your head. Keep the dumbbell above your head and take 4 seconds to lower your body to the starting position.

10 repetitions [*Advanced*]

Lower Abs

BENT-LEG KNEE RAISE

Lie on your back with your head and neck relaxed and your hands on the floor near your butt. Your feet should be flat on the floor. Use your lower abdominal muscles to raise your knees up toward your rib cage, then slowly lower your feet back to the starting position. As your feet lightly touch the floor, repeat.

12 repetitions [*Beginner*]

PULSE-UP

Lie with your hands underneath your tailbone and your legs raised and pointed straight up toward the ceiling, perpendicular to your torso. Pull your navel inward and flex your glutes as you lift your hips just a few inches off the floor. Then lower your hips.

12 repetitions [*Beginner*]

HANGING KNEE RAISE

Hang fully extended from a chinup bar, with your palms facing out and your hands a little farther than shoulder-width apart. (Your feet may lightly touch the floor.) Raise your knees toward your chest, curling your pelvis upward at the end. When you can do that for 12 repetitions, make it tougher by keeping your legs straight instead of bending your knees or by holding a medicine ball between your knees.

12 repetitions [*Beginner to intermediate*]

SEATED AB CRUNCH

Sit on the edge of a stable chair or bench. Place your hands in front of your butt and grip the sides of the seat. Lean back slightly and extend your legs down and away, keeping your heels 4 to 6 inches off the floor. To begin the exercise, bend your knees and slowly raise your legs toward your chest. At the same time, lean forward with your upper body, allowing your chest to approach your thighs.

12 repetitions [*Beginner to intermediate*]

RAISED KNEE-IN

Lie on your back. Your arms should be close to your sides, with your palms down and just under your lower back and butt. Press the small of your back against the floor and extend your legs outward, with your heels about 3 inches above the floor. Keeping your lower back against the floor, lift your left knee toward your chest. Your right leg should remain hovering above the floor. Hold, then straighten your left leg to the starting position and repeat with your right leg. Keep your abs tight throughout the exercise.

8–12 repetitions each side [*Intermediate*]

FIGURE-8 CRUNCH

Lie on your back with your knees bent at a 90-degree angle and your feet
flat on the floor. Squeeze a light medicine ball tightly between your knees.
Cup your hands lightly over your ears, then slowly raise your head,
shoulders, and feet off the floor. Move your knees in a wide figure-8
motion. Do three repetitions in one direction, then reverse the motion for
three repetitions.

6 repetitions [*Intermediate*]

FLUTTER KICK

Lie on your back, raise both feet about a foot off the ground, and scissor-kick one leg over the other.

20 repetitions [*Intermediate*]

SWISS BALL KNEE RAISE

Lie faceup on a Swiss ball, with your hips lower than your shoulders. Reach back and grab something that won't move, such as a bench or desk. Lift and bend your legs so that your feet are off the floor and the lower parts of your legs point ahead. (To make it more difficult, hold your legs straight out.) Do a standard Bent-Leg Knee Raise, using your abs and hip flexors to curl your knees toward your chest.

12 repetitions [*Intermediate to advanced*]

REVERSE CRUNCH HOLDING MEDICINE BALL

Lie on a slant board with your hips lower than your head. Grab the bar
behind your head for support. Bend your hips and knees at 90-degree
angles and hold a small medicine ball between your knees. Start with your
butt flat against the board. Pull your hips up and in toward your rib cage.
Curl them as high as you can without lifting your shoulders off the board,
and keep your hips and knees at 90-degree angles.

12 repetitions [*Intermediate to advanced*]

PUSH-AWAY

Lie on your back with your hands on your chest, legs extended, feet raised off the floor. Alternately bring each knee toward your head, then forcefully kick forward. Don't let your feet touch the floor. (If you feel any discomfort in your lower back while performing this exercise, try lifting your head and tucking your chin toward your chest.)

10 repetitions each side [*Intermediate to advanced*]

Obliques

OBLIQUE V-UP

Lie on your side with your body in a straight line. Fold your arms across your chest. Keeping your legs together, lift them off the floor as you raise your top elbow toward your hip. The range of motion is short, but you should feel an intense contraction in your obliques.

10 repetitions each side [*Beginner*]

SAXON SIDE BEND

Hold a pair of lightweight dumbbells over your head, in line with your shoulders, with your elbows slightly bent. Keep your back straight, and slowly bend directly to your left side as far as possible without twisting your upper body. Pause, return to an upright position, then bend to your right side as far as possible.

6–10 repetitions each side [*Beginner to intermediate*]

SPEED ROTATION

Stand while holding a dumbbell with both hands in front of your midsection. Twist 90 degrees to the right, then 180 degrees to your left. Keep your abs tight and move fast. Bring to center. Alternate the side you start with.

10 repetitions each side [*Intermediate*]

TWO-HANDED WOOD CHOP

Stand while holding a dumbbell, with both hands next to your right ear. Flex your abs and rotate your torso to the left as you extend your arms and lower the dumbbell to the outside of your left knee. Lift it back, finish the set, and repeat on the other side.

10 repetitions each side [*Intermediate*]

MEDICINE BALL TORSO ROTATION

Hold a medicine ball or basketball in front of you. Sit with your knees bent and your feet on the floor. Quickly twist to your left and set the ball behind your back. Twist to the right and pick up the ball. Bring the ball around to your left and set it down again. Repeat. Do the same number of repetitions in which you first twist to the left side as you do when you twist to the right side.

10 repetitions each side [*Intermediate to advanced*]

SIDE JACKKNIFE

Lie on your left hip, with your legs nearly straight and slightly raised off the floor. Also raise your torso off the floor, with your left forearm on the floor for balance. Hold your other hand behind your right ear, with your elbow pointed toward your feet. Lift your legs toward your torso while keeping your torso stationary. Pause to feel the contraction on the right side of your waist. Then slowly lower your legs and repeat. Finish the set on that side, then lie on your right hip and do the same number of repetitions.

10 repetitions each side [*Intermediate to advanced*]

Transverse Abdominis

BRIDGE

Start to get in a Pushup position, but bend your elbows and rest your weight on your forearms instead of your hands. Your body should form a straight line from your shoulders to your ankles. Pull your abdominals in; imagine you're trying to move your belly button back to your spine. Hold for 20 seconds, breathing steadily. As you build endurance, you can do one 60-second set.

1–2 repetitions [*Beginner to intermediate*]

SIDE BRIDGE

Lie on your nondominant side. Support your weight with that forearm and the outside edge of that foot. Your body should form a straight line from head to ankles. Pull your abs in as far as you can and hold this position for 10 to 30 seconds, breathing steadily. Relax. If you can do 30 seconds, do one repetition. If not, try for any combination of reps that gets you up to 30 seconds. Repeat on your other side.

1–2 repetitions each side [*Beginner to intermediate*]

TWO-POINT BRIDGE

Get into the standard Pushup position. Lift your left arm and your right leg off the floor at the same time. Hold for 3 to 5 seconds. That's one repetition. Return to the starting position, then repeat, lifting your right arm and left leg this time.

6–10 repetitions each side [*Intermediate*]

NEGATIVE CRUNCH

Sit on the floor with your knees bent and your feet flat on the floor and shoulder-width apart. Extend your arms with your fingers interlaced, palms facing your knees. Begin with your upper body at slightly less than a 90-degree angle to the floor. Lower your body toward the floor, curling your torso forward, rounding your lower back, and keeping your abs contracted. When your body reaches a 45-degree angle to the floor, return to the starting position. (Note: You may need to tuck your feet under a set of weights to help maintain balance throughout the exercise.)

10 repetitions [*Intermediate*]

SWISS BALL BRIDGE

Rest your forearms on a Swiss ball and your toes on the floor, with your body in a straight line. Pull your stomach in, trying to bring your belly button to your spine. Hold for 20 seconds, breathing steadily. As you build endurance, you can do one 60-second set.

1–2 repetitions [*Intermediate to advanced*]

SWISS BALL PULL-INS

Get into the Pushup position—your hands set slightly wider than and in line with your shoulders—but instead of placing your feet on the floor, rest your shins on a Swiss ball. With your arms straight and your back flat, your body should form a straight line from your shoulders to your ankles. Roll the ball toward your chest. Pause, then return the ball to the starting position by extending your legs and rolling the ball backward.

5–10 repetitions [*Intermediate to advanced*]

TOWEL ROLL

Kneel on a towel or mat on a tile or wooden floor. Put a towel on the floor in front of you, and place your hands on it. Slide the towel across the floor until your body is fully extended. Your body should look as if you're in a diving position. Slowly slide back up.

5–10 repetitions [*Advanced*]

BARBELL ROLLOUT

Load a pair of 5-pound plates onto a barbell. Kneel on an exercise mat or towel, with your shoulders directly over the bar. Grab the bar with an overhand, shoulder-width grip. Start with your back in a slightly rounded position, allowing it to extend into a more neutral position as you execute the movement. Roll the bar out in front of you, holding your knees in place as your hips, torso, and arms go forward. Keeping your arms taut, advance as far as you can without arching your back or touching the floor with anything above your knees. Pause for a split second, then pull back to the starting position.

5–10 repetitions [*Advanced*]

Lower Back

BACK EXTENSION

Position yourself in a back extension station and hook your feet under the leg anchor. Hold your arms straight out in front of you. Your body should form a straight line from your hands to your hips. Lower your torso, allowing your lower back to round, until it's just short of perpendicular to the floor. Raise your upper body until it's slightly above parallel to the floor. At this point, you should have a slight arch in your back, and your shoulder blades should be pulled together. Pause for a second, then repeat.

12–15 repetitions [*Beginner to intermediate*]

TWISTING BACK EXTENSION

Position yourself in a back extension station and hook your feet under the leg anchor. Place your fingers lightly behind or over your ears. Lower your upper body, allowing your lower back to round, until it's just short of perpendicular to the floor. Raise and twist your upper body until it's slightly above parallel to the floor and facing right. Pause, then lower your torso and repeat, this time twisting to the left.

12–15 repetitions [*Intermediate*]

SWISS BALL SUPERMAN

Lie facedown over a Swiss ball so that your hips are pressed against the ball and your torso is rounded over it. Lift your upper arms so that they're parallel to your body, and bend your elbows 90 degrees so that your hands are pointing forward and your elbows are pointing back. Slowly extend your back until your chest is completely off the ball, extend your arms forward, and hold that position. Draw your arms back into position as you return your torso to the ball.

12–15 repetitions [*Intermediate*]

SWIMMER'S BACKSTROKE

Lie faceup on the floor, with your knees bent and feet flat. Flatten your lower back against the floor. Now do a crunch to flex your trunk forward and lift your shoulder blades as high off the floor as you possibly can. Keeping your chest high, perform a backstroke with one arm at a time, allowing your torso to twist toward the arm that's reaching back. Work up to 5 repetitions of 45 seconds each, alternating arms. The higher you lift your chest off the floor, the better the exercise will work. Add light dumbbells when this move becomes too easy.

1–5 repetitions [*Intermediate to advanced*]

Bonus! 18 Above-the-Belt Time-Savers!

Looking to shave even more time off your workout while shaving fat from your waistline? The remaining 18 moves of our 50-"6-pack" plan work several areas of your midsection simultaneously. Use any one of the following substitutions to cover two or three areas with one exercise, and you can reduce your workout plan to just a few exercises instead of five!

CRUNCH/SIDE BEND COMBO
Targets both the upper abs and obliques
Lie on your back, with your knees bent and your hands behind your ears. Curl up so that your shoulder blades are off the floor. Bend at the waist to the left, aiming your left armpit toward your right hip. Straighten, then bend to your right.

8 repetitions each side [*Beginner*]

SINGLE-KNEE CRUNCH
Targets both the upper and lower abs

Lie on your back, with your hips bent 90 degrees and your feet flat on the floor. Touch your fingers to the sides of your head, with your elbows bent. Raise your head, shoulders, and butt off the floor as you simultaneously bring your left knee toward your chest. Lower your torso and leg back down, then repeat the exercise, this time drawing your right knee up instead as you crunch.

10 repetitions each side [*Beginner to intermediate*]

TWISTING CRUNCH
Targets both the upper abs and obliques

Lie on your back on the floor, with your hands cupped behind your ears and your elbows out. Cross your ankles, with your knees slightly bent, and raise your legs until your thighs are perpendicular to your body. Bring your right shoulder off the floor as you cross your right elbow over to your left knee. Return to the starting position and repeat, beginning with the left shoulder, crossing your left elbow over to your right knee.

8 repetitions each side [*Beginner to intermediate*]

STICK CRUNCH
Targets both the upper and lower abs

Lie on your back, with your feet raised off the ground and your knees slightly bent. Hold a broomstick behind your head, with your arms extended and off the ground. Crunch your torso up and draw your knees up so that the stick extends past your knees. Pause, then return to the starting position.

12 repetitions [*Intermediate*]

BICYCLE
Targets both the upper and lower abs

Lying on your back with your knees bent 90 degrees and your hands behind your ears, pump your legs back and forth, bicycle-style, as you rotate your torso from side to side by moving an armpit (not an elbow) toward the opposite knee.

20 repetitions [*Intermediate*]

WEIGHTED ONE-SIDED CRUNCH
Targets both the upper abs and obliques

Lie with your knees bent and feet flat on the floor. Hold a dumbbell by your left shoulder with both hands. Curl your torso up and rotate to the right. Lower yourself, finish the set, then repeat, placing the dumbbell next to your right shoulder.

8 repetitions each side [*Intermediate*]

OBLIQUE HANGING LEG RAISE
Targets both the lower abs and obliques

Grasp a chinup bar with an overhand grip and hang from it at arm's length, with your knees bent. Keep your knees bent and lift your left hip toward your left armpit until your lower legs are nearly parallel to the floor. Pause, then return to the starting position, and lift your right hip toward your right armpit.

10 repetitions each side [*Intermediate*]

HANGING SINGLE-KNEE RAISE
Targets both the lower abs and obliques

Hang fully extended from a chinup bar, with your palms facing out and your hands a little farther than shoulder-width apart. Your feet should lightly touch the floor. Without swinging to pick up momentum, raise your right knee toward your left shoulder as far as you can, using your abs for power. Slightly thrust your pelvis forward to help, but don't rock. Hold for a second, then lower to the starting position. Repeat with your left leg, raising it toward your right shoulder.

8–12 repetitions each side [*Intermediate*]

KNEELING THREE-WAY CABLE CRUNCH
Targets both the upper abs and obliques

Attach a rope to the handle of the high pulley. Kneel facing the pulley, and grab the ends of the rope, with your palms facing each other. Hold the rope along the sides of your face, with your elbows slightly bent. Bend forward at the waist, rounding your back and aiming your chest at your pelvis. Stop when you feel a contraction in your abdominal muscles. Return to the starting position, then repeat the movement, this time aiming your chest toward your right knee. Stop when you feel a contraction in your right obliques. Return, then repeat the movement to your left. That's one repetition.

8 repetitions [*Intermediate to advanced*]

RUSSIAN TWIST
Targets both the upper abs and obliques

Sit on the floor, with your knees bent and your feet flat. Hold your arms straight out in front of your chest, with your palms facing down. Lean back so that your torso is at a 45-degree angle to the floor. Twist to the right as far as you can, pause, then reverse your movement and twist all the way back to the left as far as you can. As you get stronger, hold a light weight in your hands as you do the movement. (Note: You may need to tuck your feet under a set of weights to help maintain balance throughout the exercise.)

10 repetitions each side [*Intermediate to advanced*]

V-SPREAD TOE TOUCH
Targets both the upper abs and obliques

Lie flat on your back, with your legs straight up in a V position without locking your knees. Raise your arms toward the ceiling. Curl your shoulder blades up and reach toward your right foot with both hands. Hold for a second, concentrating on your abs, then lower to the starting position. Repeat, this time reaching for your left foot. Don't pause at the lower position.

12–15 repetitions [*Intermediate to advanced*]

CORKSCREW
Targets both the lower abs and obliques

Lie on your back, with your legs raised directly over your hips; your knees should be slightly bent. Place your hands with the palms down at your sides. Use your lower abs to raise your hips off the floor and toward your rib cage, elevating your hips straight up toward the ceiling. Simultaneously twist your hips to the right in a corkscrew motion. Hold, then return to the starting position. Repeat, twisting to the left.

10 repetitions [*Intermediate to advanced*]

STRAIGHT-LEG CYCLING CRUNCH
Targets both the upper and lower abs

Lie on your back and bend your hips and knees 90 degrees so that your feet are in the air. Place your hands behind your ears and perform an abdominal crunch by lifting your head and shoulders off the floor. At the same time, lift your right leg to your chest. Lower your torso to the floor as you straighten your right leg, keeping it a few inches off the floor. Repeat the exercise, this time drawing your left knee up as you crunch. Alternate from right to left throughout the exercise.

10 repetitions each side [*Advanced*]

LATERAL MEDICINE BALL BLAST
Targets both the upper abs and obliques

Set an adjustable ab bench at a 45-degree angle. Lie down on it and hook your feet under the padded support bars. Hold a medicine ball or weight plate against your chest. As you come up, twist to the left and extend your arms as if you were throwing the ball or weight. Pull it back to your chest as you untwist and lower yourself. Repeat, twisting to the right.

5 repetitions each side [*Advanced*]

KNEE RAISE WITH DROP
Targets both the lower abs and obliques

Lie on your back, with your hands behind your ears, hips and knees bent, and feet on the floor. Position a medicine ball between your knees. Keep your lower back on the floor throughout the exercise. Contract your abdominals and pull your knees to your chest. Lower your knees to the left, bring them back to center, then return to the starting position. Drop your knees to the right on the next repetition and alternate sides for each rep.

12 repetitions [*Advanced*]

DOUBLE CRUNCH
Targets both the upper and lower abs

Lie on your back, with your hips and knees bent and your feet on the floor. Rest your hands lightly on your chest. Position a medicine ball between your knees. Exhale as you lift your shoulders off the floor and bring your knees to your chest. Grab the ball with your hands and bring it to your chest as you inhale and return your shoulders and legs to the starting position. Transfer the ball back to your legs on the next repetition and keep alternating ball positions for the entire set.

12 repetitions [*Advanced*]

V-UPS
Targets both the upper and lower abs

Lie on your back, with your legs and arms extended. Keeping your knees and elbows locked, simultaneously raise your upper body while trying to touch your fingers to your toes.

5–10 repetitions [*Advanced*]

DOUBLE CRUNCH WITH A CROSS
Targets both the upper and lower abs, plus the obliques

Lie on your back with your knees bent, your feet flat on the floor, your head and neck relaxed, and your hands behind your ears. Use your lower abs to lift both knees and cross them toward your left shoulder as you simultaneously use your upper abs to raise your left shoulder and cross it toward your right knee. Hold for a second. Lower your legs and torso to the starting position and repeat to the other side.

10 repetitions each side [*Advanced*]

THE SECRET TO LEAN LEGS

Lower-Body Toning and Shaping Exercises for Your Abs Diet Workout

s you've learned, getting a flat belly is not only about doing exercises that work and strengthen your midsection. It's also about working your whole body so you build a critical mass of lean muscle that will help you burn fat. The best fat burner of all: your leg muscles. Because they're so big, you can chew up a lot of fat by adding some muscle to them. Added bonus: You'll tone and firm them at the same time. And what woman doesn't want leaner, firmer, more shapely butt, thighs, and calves? Take a look at some leg-specific variations you can substitute or add into your Abs Diet Circuit.

STRETCH IT OUT

If your hamstrings are tight, you may develop a habit of leaning backward to relieve the pressure. This tends to thrust your gut forward, making you look paunchy. Stretching your hamstrings a few times a week should help. The fastest, easiest way to loosen up your back and hamstrings and tighten your abs is by doing the Figure-4 Stretch. Sit on the floor with your right leg straight in front of you, toes pointing up. Bend your left knee to place your left heel against the inside of your right thigh, near your groin; keep your left knee almost touching the floor. Now reach out slowly with your right arm and touch your right ankle or toe. Hold for 30 seconds, return to the starting position, and then repeat. Switch legs and stretch your left side twice also.

Lunges

The lunge is the ultimate all-in-one lower-body exercise—it works your thighs, hamstring, and glutes, and it also works your abs and core because you need those muscles to stabilize yourself while you're on one leg. These lunges will add some variety to your workout if you sub them in for the squat or traveling lunge in the Abs Diet Circuit.

LUNGE WITH UPRIGHT ROW
Works legs, shoulders, and upper back
Hold a pair of 5-pound dumbbells and let your arms hang in front of you, palms facing your body. Next, step the right leg into a lunge, while simultaneously pulling your hands up your body until your elbows are even with your shoulders. Lower your arms and return to start. Repeat with your left leg and alternate sides for 12 reps.

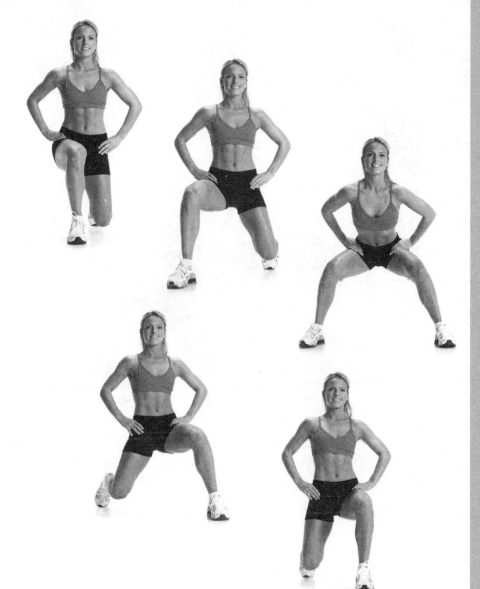

PENTA LUNGE
Strengthens legs and glutes from every angle
Step forward with your right foot into a regular lunge. Next, push back and lunge out 45 degrees to the right (in front of you). Then lunge to the right side, push up, and lunge 45 degrees behind you. Finish by stepping back into a regular reverse lunge. Repeat with the left leg and alternate for each sequence.

STEP LUNGE PULSE
Tones thighs and glutes

Stand in front of a step (or Bosu or foam pad) and step onto it, placing your left foot flat on top. Sink your weight down into a lunge. Keeping your foot on the step, press up and then sink down again for another rep. Perform 10 reps and then switch sides.

LUNGE KICK AND CURL
Works legs, glutes, and biceps

Grab two dumbbells and step your right leg back into a reverse lunge. As you press up, kick your back leg in front while curling the dumbbells toward your shoulders. Step your right leg back into a reverse lunge and repeat. Do 10 reps before switching legs.

OVERHEAD LUNGE WALK
Strengthens legs, glutes, core, and shoulders

Hold a light barbell or two dumbbells at arm's length over your head, palms facing forward. Pull your abs in toward your spine to stabilize your core. Step your right leg forward into a lunge, then press up and step forward into a lunge with your left leg. Keep walking for 10 lunges.

FLAMINGO LUNGE
Works legs, shoulders, chest, and triceps

Hold a medicine ball in front of your chest at shoulder height. Step back with your right foot into a reverse lunge. As you push up to start, press the ball over your head as you lift your right leg in front, bending your right knee to 90 degrees. Balance for a second. Lower the weight and repeat on the same leg for 10 reps. Then repeat with your left leg.

Vary Nice Legs

As it goes with most basic exercises: You can make adjustments and tweaks to them to challenge your body even more as you become fitter and stronger. With these three exercises, use Level 1 as the foundation. Once you've mastered them, you can progress to Levels 2 (pages 291 to 293) and 3 (pages 294 to 296) to add in variety. Sub them in for lunges, squats, or step-ups in the Abs Diet Circuit.

LEVEL 1 MOVES

SQUAT

Hold a barbell with an overhand grip so that it rests comfortably on your upper back. Set your feet about shoulder width apart, and keep your knees slightly bent, back straight, and eyes focused straight ahead. Slowly lower your body as if you were sitting back into a chair, keeping your back in its natural alignment and your lower legs nearly perpendicular to the floor. Don't let your knees move forward over your toes. Don't round your back. Stop just before your thighs are parallel to the floor. Hold for a second and then exhale as you slowly stand back up.

BACK LUNGE

Stand with your feet together and place your hands on your hips. Step your right foot back 2 to 3 feet. Inhale as you bend your left knee and lower your body straight down until your left knee is bent 90 degrees and your right knee nearly touches the floor. Your rear heel will come off the floor. Don't lean forward. Don't let your front knee move forward over your toes. Hold for a second and then exhale as you push yourself back up, bringing your right foot in. Finish all of your repetitions, then repeat the exercise stepping your left foot back.

STEP SQUAT

Stand with your feet together and your hands down at your sides. Step your left foot out to the side 2 to 2½ feet. Keeping your back straight, lower yourself, bending from the knees and hips as though you're sitting down, as you inhale. Let your arms come out in front of you to help you balance. Stop just before your thighs are parallel to the floor. Don't let your knees move forward over your toes. Don't round your back. Hold for a second and then exhale as you push back up, bringing your left foot back in. Do five or six reps with your left foot, and then do five or six reps stepping with your right foot.

LEVEL 2 MOVES

PLIÉ SQUAT

Stand with your feet wider than shoulder-width apart, toes pointing out. Hold a dumbbell with both hands down in front of you. Keeping your back straight, lower yourself, bending from your knees, as you inhale. Stop just before your thighs are parallel to the floor. Don't let your knees move forward over your toes. Don't lean forward. Hold for a second and then exhale as you slowly stand back up.

BACK LUNGE WITH KNEE LIFT

Stand with your feet together. Hold a dumbbell in each hand, either at shoulder height or at your sides. Step your right foot back 2 to 3 feet. Inhale as you bend your left knee and lower your body straight down until your left knee is bent 90 degrees and your right knee nearly touches the floor. Your rear heel will come off the floor. Don't lean forward. Don't let your front knee move forward over your toes. Hold for a second and then exhale as you push yourself back up. Lift your right knee up in front of you before bringing it back to the starting position. Finish all of your repetitions, then repeat the exercise, stepping back with your left foot.

STEP SQUAT WITH KNEE LIFT

Stand with your feet together. Hold a dumbbell in each hand, either at shoulder height or at your sides. Step your left foot out to the side 2 to 2½ feet. Keeping your back straight, lower yourself, bending from the knees and hips as you inhale. Stop just before your thighs are parallel to the floor. Don't let your knees move forward over your toes. Don't round your back. Hold for a second and then exhale as you push back up, lifting your left knee out in front of you before returning to the starting position. Do five or six reps with your left foot and then do five or six reps stepping with your right foot.

LEVEL 3 MOVES

ONE-LEG SQUAT

Hold dumbbells in each hand at shoulder height or down at your sides. Shift your weight to your left foot and lift your right foot off the floor so that only your toes are lightly touching for balance. As you inhale, bend your left knee and lean forward slightly from your hips, lowering yourself as if you were sitting in a chair. Go as low as is comfortable, but don't go past your left thigh being parallel to the floor. Don't let your working knee come forward past your toes. Hold for a second and then exhale as you slowly stand back up. Do the recommended number of reps and then switch legs.

FRONT LUNGE WITH JUMP

Stand with your feet together and your arms at your sides. Step your right foot forward 2 to 3 feet. Inhale as you bend your right knee and lower your body straight down until your right knee is bent 90 degrees and your left knee nearly touches the floor. Your rear heel will come off the floor. Don't lean forward. Don't let your front knee move forward over your toes. Hold for a second and then exhale as you push off with your right foot and jump your feet together. Finish all of your repetitions, then repeat the exercise, stepping forward with your left foot.

STEP SQUAT WITH JUMP

Stand with your feet together and your hands down at your sides. Don't do this move while holding weights. Step your left foot out to the side 2 to 2½ feet. Keeping your back straight, lower yourself, bending from the knees and hips as though you're sitting down, as you inhale. Let your arms come out in front of you to help you balance. Stop just before your thighs are parallel to the floor. Don't let your knees move forward over your toes. Don't round your back. Hold for a second and then exhale as you jump and bring your left foot back in next to your right foot. Do five or six reps with your left foot and then do five or six reps stepping with your right foot.

The One-Move Workout!

Crunched for time? At the very least, you can do an exercise that works many of your major muscles at once. The move shown below works almost all of your big muscles simultaneously, so you burn more calories per rep. It also strengthens your whole core, so you'll have better balance and stability and be less prone to lower-back injuries.

Hold a dumbbell with both hands in front of your body and raise it up over your head as you pivot on your right foot and rotate your body to the left, lifting the dumbbell up over your left shoulder. Lower your body and chop the dumbbell down toward your right foot, allowing your feet to pivot. You'll end up in a lunge position. Rotate back to the left, lifting your body and bringing the dumbbell back up. Repeat for 10 reps before switching sides. Add some variation with these three changes.

▶ Go faster: If you speed up your pace, it will force your core to work harder to stabilize your body as you squat, twist, and lift.

▶ Extend your reach: By reaching out more over your toe (and extending farther over your shoulder), you'll add more leverage to the exercise and increase your range of motion.

▶ Get heavy: Heavier weight equals heavier sweat.

Chapter **16**

THE ABS DIET AND YOUR HORMONES
How the Program Can Work with Your Body's Natural Cycles

SAY THE WORD *HORMONES* TO A MAN and the only thing he thinks about is the next time he's going to indulge his. But say the word to a woman, and she understands the complexity, the nuances, and the power that her hormones have. They control moods, they control reproduction, and they can control whether you burn fat or store it.

Though they often seem to be unleashed like a pit bull in a butcher shop, hormones can be kept under control—if you know what to do. Research shows that there are many things you can do to keep your hormones functioning at normal levels, whether you're experiencing natural drops in estrogen that happen during the aging process or you're having trouble burning fat because of a thyroid hormone that's fritzing out like your aunt's 1973 TV set. These strategies will help you manage the fluctuating hormone levels you may be experiencing, all while adopting the Abs Diet as your new, fat-burning, body-changing lifestyle.

Beat PMS

POPPING OTC medication isn't the only thing you can do to help alleviate the cramps, foul moods, and hunger that come with the fluctuating levels of estrogen and progesterone you experience before your period. Try these easy lifestyle changes that can ease some of the cyclical burden.

▶ Even more than you usually do on the Abs Diet, focus on eating protein and fiber to keep your blood sugar even, slow your rate of digestion, and resist the urge to overeat. The best foods include whole grains, fruits, and vegetables.

▶ A University of Massachusetts at Amherst study found that a high intake of calcium and vitamin D decreases the severity of PMS symptoms, plus it prevents PMS from initially developing. The study concluded that women who ate or drank about 1,200 milligrams of calcium and 400 IU of vitamin D daily had significantly lower risk of developing PMS. That's the equivalent of four servings a day of fat-free or low-fat milk, other low-fat dairy products like yogurt, or fortified orange juice.

▶ Have the perfect breakfast. It combines vitamin B_6 with magnesium (both found in salmon and avocados), two nutrients that have been shown to relieve monthly mood swings. This magical meal also includes cheese, which helps replenish the vitamin D and calcium that your period can deplete. And it features fiber: A high-fiber diet has been shown to ease PMS symptoms by expelling excess estrogen. Best, it includes three Powerfoods! Here's the secret recipe.

2   slices 100 percent whole-grain bread, toasted

1   tablespoon low-fat cream cheese

¼   avocado

1   ounce smoked salmon

    Freshly ground pepper

    Small handful of alfalfa sprouts or fresh spinach

On one slice of toast, spread the cheese and layer the avocado and fish. Top with the pepper, sprouts, and second slice of toast.

▶ You can cut down on period-related migraines and headaches associated with drops in estrogen levels by eliminating foods that tend to trigger them. The most common foods include aged cheeses, processed meats with nitrates, chocolate, excessive caffeine, alcohol (especially red wine), citrus foods, bananas, aspartame, and MSG. Exercise and meditation also seem to help reduce the risk of developing migraines, partly because they reduce stress (a migraine trigger).

▶ A yoga pose that opens up the pelvic area can relieve bloating and cramps. Try a pose called Reclining Bound Angle. To do it, sit on the floor with a long pillow behind you. The bottom should touch your sacrum, and a folded blanket should cover the top. Lie back into the pillow, resting your head on the blanket. Put the soles of your feet together and let your knees and thighs fall to the sides. Stay in the pose for 5 to 10 minutes and breathe deeply.

▶ A recent study found that taking 200 IU of vitamin E twice daily 2 days before—and 3 days during—menstruation can ease cramps. Those in the study who took the vitamin E experienced fewer than 2 hours of cramps per cycle, down from 17 on average. And only 4 percent of the women needed a pain reliever for cramp relief. The theory is that vitamin E hinders the formation of prostaglandins, the hormonelike chemicals that cause uterine contractions. But take E only for those 5 prescribed days each month; high doses taken over years at a time have been linked to heart trouble.

▶ Ask your doctor about tweaking your birth control regimen. In a Yale study, oral contraceptives reduced PMS symptoms by 50 percent in half the participants using 24 hormone pills and 4 sugar pills.

▶ Acupressure may also help ease symptoms. Research suggests that acupressure stimulates bloodflow and releases endorphins—the body's natural painkillers. In one study, those who had acupressure had 72 percent less pain (the same as those who took ibuprofen), while those who had a false acupressure treatment (not performed on the correct spots) had a 58 percent decrease.

Manage Menopause

LIFE IS FULL of transitions. You start a new job or watch your kids go off to kindergarten or adjust to a new season of *Survivor*. When it comes to her health, every woman has to deal with at least one major—and natural—transition. From a purely scientific standpoint, menopause—which usually occurs between ages 40 and 55—is defined as the period of time when a woman's ovaries stop producing eggs and her body ceases production of two major hormones: estrogen and progesterone (perimenopause is the start of these hormonal changes).

The outward sign is that menstruation becomes less and less frequent until it stops altogether. But it's also defined by many other signs because of the symptoms associated with the changing hormonal levels. These symptoms occur as your body finds ways to rebel against the declining hormonal levels.

Like a good bouillabaisse, all women aren't made the same way—especially when it comes to how they respond to menopause. While some women have mild symptoms, others have very severe responses; the severity of symptoms is usually caused by how suddenly or slowly the ovaries slow hormone production. The most common symptoms—everything from hot flashes, insomnia, mood swings, vaginal dryness, infections, and a loss of sex drive—can also be accompanied by longer-term changes that can lead to such things as bone loss and higher cholesterol levels. Because menopause is a normal and natural aging process, it's not something you try to treat or prevent the way you would heart disease or cancer. Instead, your goal is to lessen the severity of the symptoms associated with it. Fortunately, there are many things that you can do naturally to decrease both the severity of symptoms and the risk of other problems that stem from menopause.

Use the Abs Diet to keep your weight down. In the Iowa Women's Health Study, researchers found that the risk of breast cancer for postmenopausal women was 44 percent higher for those who weighed more. The high-risk group had a body mass index of 29.5 or higher, while the low-risk group had a BMI of 23.5 or lower (page 58 showed you how to calculate your BMI). Related to that, another study found that maintaining weight helps reduce the risk of coronary problems in post-menopausal women. And that's important: A recent study of more than 60,000 women found that 17 percent had a moderate to high likelihood of having a silent heart attack (that's a heart attack with no noticeable symptoms). It's particularly important to keep an eye on your weight because this is an especially difficult time; one animal study showed that body weight can jump up 5 percent during menopause.

Bear fruit. Some fruits and vegetables contain phytoestrogens—elements that may trick the body into thinking it has higher levels of estrogen, which can help ease symptoms. Fruits with high phytoestrogens include plums, strawberries, apples, grapes, oranges, and raspberries. Vegetables include asparagus, cauliflower, broccoli, carrots, cucumbers, onions, and soybeans.

Go fish. Fish high in omega-3 fatty acids help add good cholesterol, which can help reduce the risk of heart attack (remember, it increases after menopause). You can also sub in flaxseed for additional omega-3s.

Embrace fat. Eating a small amount of dietary fat in one sitting can stimulate the gallbladder to empty, which helps prevent gallstones—which can be more common in menopause. Think almonds.

Go out shopping. And walk the aisles. A review of studies published in the journal *Sports Medicine* found that walking 30 minutes every day and one to three bouts of resistance training a week improved the health-related fitness of early postmenopausal women. The researchers determined the ranges by looking at the impact of various activities on bone mineral density, balance, insulin sensitivity, cholesterol, and body composition. Exercise may also help reduce menopausal symptoms by releasing endorphins—natural antidepressants that can help reduce incidences of insomnia, depression, mood swings, and headaches.

Huff. Though you may associate hot flashes with getting a glimpse of Usher's abs, they're more common in menopausal women for another reason. They occur because declining hormonal levels cause your internal thermostat to become unstable, making your body feel too hot. To cool down, blood vessels dilate and send a rush of blood to the surface of the skin—typically around your face, neck, and upper body. Your skin will get hot, you may sweat, and you may feel a prickly sensation during one of these flashes, which can last anywhere from 5 to 15 minutes. Hot flashes can cause all kinds of other symptoms, including insomnia and irritability. But you can decrease the effects of a hot flash with slow breathing exercises—go for slow, controlled breaths that last 10 seconds.

Keep a journal. As you enter perimenopause, you'll want to record information about your periods to note any irregularities in terms of flow or duration. But it's also smart to keep track of things that happen when you have hot flashes; you may find that you can identify the triggers—whether it's alcohol, spicy food, or hot weather—so you can figure out alternatives to avoid them.

Cohosh b'gosh. Black cohosh—an alternative remedy—has been shown in some studies to be effective at treating hot flashes.

Add water. As estrogen decreases in your body, you may experience vaginal dryness—increasing the chance of painful sex and decreasing the chance that you'll even want to make love. Water-based lubricants like Astroglide can help (avoid oil-based ones, which can actually dry out vaginal tissue).

Thyroid Hormone: The Metabolism-Busting Hormone

AS YOU'VE PROBABLY figured out by now, there's a lot that goes into how your metabolism works—through what you eat and how you move. But eating sufficient protein and choosing a walk at lunch over Popeye's aren't the only things that control your metabolic rate. Your genetics plays a large part, too. As much as you can control your metabolism through your foods and exercise, you're not the sole controller of your metabolic odometer. Think of your metabolism as a little bit like an electric mixer: You have a very fast speed, a very slow speed, and lots of little speeds in between. That rate of mixing—or in your case, the rate at which you burn calories—varies a lot depending on how you control it. But your body also can short out—causing your calorie-mixer to go haywire or short out altogether. In a lot of ways, that controller comes in the form of your thyroid gland—a hormone-producing gland located in the front of your neck.

Your thyroid gland is like the new puppy of your body; it gets blamed for everything that can go wrong. Your thyroid gland doesn't just regulate metabolism; it also controls things like body temperature. But if something inside your body is causing your thyroid to malfunction, it throws off all of the systems it controls. That's where hyper- and hypothyroidism can affect your metabolism and how quickly or slowly you burn calories. Hypothyroidism is a condition in which the gland fails to produce enough thyroid hormone, meaning that your metabolism can grind to a crawl and lead to weight gain or at least make it very difficult to lose weight. Hyperthyroidism is the exact opposite. It's a condition where the gland overproduces thyroid hormone, so it increases metabolism to a point where you lose weight too fast (yes, there is such a thing). The added trouble is that thyroid hormone is also linked to the pituitary gland—meaning that any kind of problems in the production of thyroid hormone can also have an effect on brain functions that involve the pituitary. That's why thyroid troubles are often difficult to diagnose. Symptoms of hypothyroidism can come in the form of slow speech, abnormal menstrual periods, muscle pain, joint stiffness, drowsiness, swelling, and a host of others, while hyperthyroidism is marked by such things as rapid weight loss, intolerance to heat, restlessness, fatigue, sleeping trouble, and other symptoms.

It's also important to understand that your weight isn't the only thing your thyroid gland can mess up. One study showed that hypothyroidism increased the odds of heart disease by 70 percent and more than doubled the odds of a heart attack. That's why it's especially essential to have regular blood tests that can measure your levels of thyroid hormone. If the doctors determine your hormonal levels are off, they can prescribe medications to help put hormone levels back at a normal range.

Chapter 17

THE ABS DIET FOR MOMS

Using the Plan to Prepare for the Baby—
And Lose the Baby Weight

IT'S TRUE: SOME PEOPLE CARRY BASKETBALL-SIZE bellies because of Death by Chocolate desserts and too many nosedives into the cheese fondue. But others carry big bellies because they're performing the single most important job in the world—carrying a child. Now, just because having a baby turns flat stomachs into bulbous ones doesn't mean that you should abandon a healthy eating and exercise lifestyle. In fact, it's even more important to maintain healthy habits before, during, and after pregnancy for your health and shape and that of your child. Just consider this study: Swedish researchers analyzed the weight of 563 women before, during, and 15 years after their pregnancies. They found that those who gained more than 35 pounds while expecting were 2½ times more likely to keep the weight after birth. You want to shoot for a gain of between 25 and 35 pounds (that's the healthy range outlined by the American College of Obstetricians and Gynecologists). And studies show that being overweight while carrying a baby increases your risk of pregnancy-related problems like gestational diabetes, preeclampsia, and Caesarean delivery.

Now, just because you'll lose your visible abs once you become pregnant doesn't mean the Abs Diet has to disappear as well. It's always vital for pregnant women to consult their doctors about any eating and exercise programs, but these are strategies for how the Abs Diet can be built for two.

Before Getting Pregnant . . .

Drop your weight. Being overweight or obese raises your risk of gestational diabetes and therefore your child's risk of heart problems and birth defects. Gestational diabetes is also linked to abnormally large babies and difficult labor. Getting to a healthy weight is also important if you're considering in vitro fertilization (IVF). If you're 30 percent above your ideal weight while undergoing IVF, your odds of having a successful pregnancy are low. In one study, obese women were 32 percent less likely to get pregnant than were women with healthy weights. Researchers suspect that losing just 5 percent of body weight can improve odds—all the more reason to commit to the Abs Diet.

Watch the carbs. Refined carbs such as soda, cookies, fruit drinks, pretzels, and white bread may increase your baby's risk of birth defects. In a March of Dimes study, those who ate the largest amounts of refined carbohydrates during the 3 months before conception doubled the threat to their babies, compared with women who ate the least. Researchers suspect that starchy or sugary foods raise a woman's blood glucose, which can lead to cell damage and deplete the fetus of a chemical messenger between cells. The fix: Powerfoods like whole grains, beans, and fruits and vegetables.

Exercise hard. A powerful incentive to do your high-intensity intervals: Researchers at the University of Washington who surveyed 688 mothers found that those who performed the most vigorous exercise during the year before pregnancy were 81 percent less likely to develop gestational diabetes than those who were sedentary, while moderate exercisers had a 59 percent lower risk.

Take folic acid. Take 400 micrograms of folic acid to help prevent birth defects, unless your multivitamin covers that amount. Be careful, though—the Food and Nutrition Board sets the safe upper limit for the nutrient at 1,000 micrograms. Good dietary sources include leafy green vegetables like spinach and fortified cereals.

Get a blood sugar check. It needs to be at a healthy level for 3 to 6 months before conception because unhealthy levels lead to increased risk of birth defects. If you have a family history of diabetes or are overweight, you're more at risk.

During Pregnancy . . .

Keep working out. Now, I'm not saying you should be signing up for marathons or trying your first 5-day adventure race, but exercising is important throughout pregnancy to maintain control of your weight as well as your tone. If you're a runner, you can keep running early in your pregnancy, but swimming is thought to be the safest cardiovascular exercise because it helps maintain body tone without stressing the joints. The one significant change you'll want to make to the Abs Diet program is to eliminate the interval workout. Doctors recommend that you keep your heart rate away from high-intensity levels. They recommend levels at which you can exercise and hold conversations at the same time—to ensure you don't overdo it. New research shows that physical activity can also make you less likely to deliver early.

Follow the Abs Diet Power 12. Though you need only 300 or so extra calories during the second and third trimesters, you need more of the food's nutrients to pass along. The recommended daily diet includes two to three servings of calcium-rich foods, three to five servings of vegetables, two to four of fruit, six to 11 of whole grains, and two to three of lean meats and other protein sources. (More below on specific nutrients.) Hmmm, by my count, that's the D, S, R, W, and T of ABS DIET POWER. Experts also recommend taking a multivitamin to ensure you're getting 400 micrograms of folic acid and calcium—the folic acid to protect against birth defects and the calcium to ensure you're getting enough to protect your bones. (The baby can take calcium away from your bones, leaving you at greater risk of osteoporosis.) Some specific recommendations:

▶ Calcium: Make sure you get at least 1,000 milligrams of calcium a day, about 200 milligrams more than before you were pregnant. An 8-ounce glass of milk has about 300 milligrams.

Your doctor may prescribe or recommend a particular supplement; if not, Citracal is a reputable choice.

▶ Iron: The National Academy of Sciences suggests you get 27 milligrams of iron daily—9 more than before you were pregnant. This will likely require a supplement because a serving of beef—one of the best iron sources—contains only 3.5 milligrams.

▶ Protein: During pregnancy you'll need about 70 grams of protein a day. That's 20 more than usual. An additional ounce of cheese or serving of meat is enough.

Stick to six. Just because you're eating for two doesn't mean you can eat around the clock. If you get your six well-balanced meals, you'll be getting enough calories and nutrients for both of you. One interesting side note about what your baby needs: A study in the *British Medical Journal* reported on an experiment done on the dietary intake of 244 pregnant women in Boston. According to the researchers, pregnant

THE MOTHER OF ALL STATISTICS

The average woman puts on 30 pounds while pregnant. Where it all goes:

▶ Baby: 7.5

▶ Placenta: 1.5

▶ Amniotic fluid: 2

▶ Uterus: 2

▶ Breasts: 2

▶ Bodily fluids: 4

▶ Maternal stores of fat, protein, and other nutrients: 7

▶ Body parts, besides the belly, that temporarily increase by one full size: bust and feet

▶ Excluding the baby's weight, pounds lost immediately after delivery: 11

women carrying males have a 10 percent higher energy intake than those carrying females. The male embryos ate 8 percent more protein, 9 percent more carbohydrates, 11 percent more animal fats, and 15 percent more vegetable fats. (See, even at an early age, we're trying to swipe stuff off your plate.) Researchers aren't sure why, but they speculate it could be caused by increased testosterone.

Now, if you're craving 16 meals a day instead of six, your best option is to try to combat cravings with handy, healthy snacks. Low-fat yogurt, low-fat cheese cubes, and baby carrots can help fend off some cravings, while dried fruit like apricots and raisins can help with a sweet pang. One really good option: Make small bags of homemade trail mix with nuts, granola, and a few pieces of dark chocolate. They'll help satisfy your sweet, salty, and crunchy cravings while also helping fill you up so you're less likely to gorge before your next meal. And if you're longing to down a tub of ice cream, you can satisfy the sweet tooth by having a cup of reduced-fat hot chocolate; it satisfies your chocolate urge, but its taste is lasting and the effect is satisfying since it takes a little longer to get through than, say, a candy bar.

Stay focused on fiber. University of Washington research shows that eating 21 grams of fiber a day lowers the risk of preeclampsia (the dangerous blood pressure condition) by about 70 percent, compared with eating less than 12 grams a day. Researchers attribute it to fiber's ability to lower blood pressure and cholesterol. You'll reach that mark by eating 2 cups of fruit, 2½ cups of vegetables, and three servings of whole grains.

Adjust your position. If you do yoga poses (as in Chapter 18), you should make slight adjustments to avoid putting your body in uncomfortable positions. Pass on postures that require you to contract or twist your abs, to avoid undue strain to the area, as well as poses that require you to lie on your belly. For standing poses, you might need to widen your stance to give your belly a little more room.

Consider ginger for nausea. Studies show that ginger is effective for relieving nausea and vomiting during pregnancy. Other studies show that ginger is as effective as vitamin B_6 for effectively reducing severe nausea.

After You Give Birth . . .

Go back to your abs workout after doctor's clearance. After you give birth, you may think your belly has reached the point of no return. But there are plenty of women who are able to regain their shape after pregnancy. It just takes a little longer. See, pregnancy stretches and weakens your abdominal muscles (C-sections weaken them even more). And it's not uncommon for some of the connective tissue around those abdominal muscles to take a year or more to return to its original strength. Ab exercises in any form work the muscles around your core to tighten and firm the entire area, and experts recommend exercises like Pilates and crunches to speed up the process. (You should always talk to your doctor about when it's safe for you to resume your workouts after childbirth.)

To start back slowly, try this exercise, which you can do while driving, sitting on the couch, or at your desk. Keeping your back supported, inhale and let your abdomen expand outward. Now exhale, drawing your abdominal muscles in, trying to bring your belly button toward your spine. Hold for a count of 30 (keep breathing). Then squeeze 10 times, pulling your belly button toward your spine with each contraction. Do it three times a day. By the way, your skin will go through similar changes as your muscles. But loose skin around the belly isn't a permanent problem. Skin is like an elastic band. When you stretch it, it'll eventually go back into shape. Tightening up postpregnancy skin takes some time, but with those same ab-strengthening exercises, it can return to prepregnancy firmness. For a complete postpartum workout, see page 312.

Join a support group. New moms who attended 12 weekly diet and exercise education sessions lost an average of 16 pounds after a year, while those who attended a single educational session lost only 3 pounds, according to a Saint Louis University study. Check with your local hospital or community center to see if they have a postpartum weight loss class.

Have your thyroid checked. Up to 10 percent of all women suffer from postpartum thyroiditis, or a decline in thyroid levels after giving birth. That may mean your metabolism will slow down and you'll hold on to weight. Ask your doctor for a thyroid test if you are gaining weight, are really tired, or have joint and muscle aches. The right medications will put your metabolism back on track.

Breastfeed if possible. Yes, nursing is one of nature's greatest forms of exercise—it burns up to 500 calories a day. And a Cornell study shows that because of that calorie burn, women who breastfed for a year after giving birth were 2.6 pounds lighter than women who didn't. It also has weight-related benefits to your child. German research found that the longer a person was breastfed during infancy, the lower that person's risk of being overweight later in life. And the rates decreased for every month that the person was breastfed—with odds of being overweight being 32 percent lower for those were breast-fed more than 9 months, compared with those who were breastfed for less than a month.

But don't rely on breastfeeding to do all the work. While it's true that nursing burns calories, the results are not the same for every-one. In fact, 20 percent of nursing moms don't lose weight. Here are some specific things to watch out for while you're nursing.

▶ To avoid a drop in your milk volume, consume at least 1,800 calories a day. Just ditch foods that don't deliver nutritionally. Avoid calorie cutting for the first month after giving birth.

▶ Nursing moms need 1,000 milligrams of calcium and at least 200 IU of vitamin D every day from food and supplements to keep their bones healthy.

▶ Eat at least three servings of low-fat dairy and five servings of fruits and vegetables daily to avoid losing out on key nutri-ents. Note that some babies are allergic to the proteins in the cow's milk that their mothers consume. Most will lose the allergy symptoms (such as green stools or eczema) when their mothers eliminate dairy products. If this is your situation, you should consult your ob-gyn on the best way to ensure you're getting enough calcium.

Be patient. Getting your body back into shape after pregnancy is surely a postpartum stressor, but Johns Hopkins researchers say that most mothers get back their prepregnancy fitness levels just a few months after delivery. The researchers found that, no matter their fitness levels or BMIs, moms returned to their prepregnancy size within 27 weeks. Though their activities may have changed, their amount of activity stayed the same (less kickboxing, more walking with jog strollers).

The Postpartum Workout

AS I SAID, when you want to resume your workouts after childbirth, you need to ask your doctor about when you can start back up, how much you can do, and what intensity is best. Most likely, she'll tell you to work your way back in slowly—heck, you've just been through nature's most intense workout ever. To ease back into your Abs Diet workouts, start with a little resistance exercise without using much weight at all. This workout will hit all of your major body parts without too much strain, and it will also serve as the signal to your body that you're ready to get back into action.

TRADITIONAL CRUNCH

Lie on your back with your knees bent and your hands behind your ears. Slowly crunch up, bringing your shoulder blades off the ground. Hold this position for 3 seconds, then return to the starting position. Do 10 repetitions. Each week, increase by one the number of crunches you perform and the number of seconds you hold each crunch.

PELVIC TILT

Lie on your back with your knees bent and your feet flat on the floor. Inhale as you raise your buttocks and contract your abs.

Hold for 5 seconds, then slowly lower, feeling each vertebra make contact with the floor. Repeat 10 times, increasing by two per week.

INNER THIGH LIFT

Lie on your left side, supporting yourself on your left elbow. Position your right hand in front of your body. Bend your right knee and position your right foot behind your left knee. Raise your left leg as high as you can, keeping your toes pointed. Slowly lower your leg. Repeat the motion, this time flexing your foot forward. Do the exercise 10 times, alternating between pointed toes and flexed foot (five times each). Then switch sides. Increase the number of repetitions you do by two each week.

PUSHUP

Get in a Pushup position with your hands about shoulder-width apart. Bend at the elbows while keeping your back straight, until your chin almost touches the floor, then push back up.

If this is too difficult, try it with your knees bent. Inhale as you raise your upper body, keeping your knees on the floor. Exhale as you lower your body. Do 10 repetitions, increasing the number of reps by two per week.

SUPERMOM

Lie flat on the floor with your legs straight and arms extended in front of you. Without moving your legs, slowly lift your torso up off the floor as high as you comfortably can, like Supermom flying off to comfort her crying baby. Pause, then lower yourself back to the floor. Do 10 repetitions, increasing the number of reps by two per week.

FIRE HYDRANT

Kneel with your hands, forearms, and elbows on the floor.
Inhale and raise your right leg out to the side, keeping your knee bent, until your thigh is parallel with the floor. Exhale as you return to the starting position. Do 10 repetitions, then switch sides. Increase the number of repetitions by two per week.

BENCH DIP

Stand with your back to a bench or chair and place your hands on the edge, fingers pointing toward your lower back. Place your feet on a chair a few feet in front of you. Keeping your hands in place, slowly step forward until your legs are entended in front of you, knees slightly bent. Your arms should be straight, elbows unlocked, supporting your weight. Slowly bend your arms to lower yourself as far as you can and bring your butt as close to the floor as possible. Press yourself back up to the starting position. Do 10 repetitions, increasing the number of reps by two per week.

SQUAT

Holding a dumbbell in each hand, stand with your feet shoulder-width apart, and keep your knees slightly bent, back straight, arms at your sides, and eyes focused straight ahead. Slowly lower your body as if you were sitting back into a chair, keeping your back in its natural alignment and your lower legs nearly perpendicular to the floor. When your thighs are parallel to the floor, pause, then return to the starting position. Do 10 repetitions, increasing the number of reps by two per week.

FORWARD STRETCH

Sit on the floor with your legs and arms stretched out in front of you. Exhale as you reach for your ankles or calves, bending your torso forward and leaning over your thighs. Hold for 10 to 15 seconds, then inhale as you return to an upright position. Repeat three times. Work up to 20 to 30 seconds per stretch and five repetitions.

Chapter 18

THE STRESS-BUSTING WORKOUT

A Program That Can Give You the Fit Body— And Calm Mind—You Want

THESE DAYS, EVERYTHING IS JUDGED BY HOW fast it can be. Fast food. Speed dating. Olympic athletes. Digital cameras. Internet connections. We're a society that's moving faster than autobahn traffic—no speed limits, just cover as much ground as you can as fast as you can. With all that we have to do, all the people we have to take care of, and all the responsibilities we have, we're always on the move—trying to squeeze every second with work, family, and, if we're lucky, a little bit of fun. What's that mean? That our brains are packed like a 5 o'clock subway, and sometimes we just crave the one thing that we can't get—the opportunity to step back.

And.

Slow.

Down.

Hey, I know you always have a lot on your plate (and it better be two or three Powerfoods!), but I also know the value of taking time for yourself to relax and recharge. One of the best ways you can slow your mind (and work your body at the same time) is through classes like yoga and Pilates. Softer and slower in pace, they can help relieve stress and, when done to supplement your Abs Diet Workout, still give you a challenging enough workout throughout the week to add calorie burn, muscle tone, and increased muscle flexibility. More and more evidence is showing the value of these kinds of workouts, no matter where you do them. For one, researchers at Jefferson Medical College took blood samples from yoga novices during a week when they took a 50-minute class. The results: Their levels of cortisol (the stress hormone) dropped immediately—even as soon as the first day of class.

And there's also evidence that yoga isn't just a spa sport anymore. In a University of Pittsburgh study, researchers put 59 obese, inactive women on a low-fat diet. Everyone walked for 40 minutes a day 5 days a week, but a third of the women did additional strength training, and another third added a yoga routine 3 days a week. After 4 months, the yogis dropped an average of 27 pounds—7 more than the walking-only group. (The strength group lost 23.)

In this chapter, I'll outline a few moves that you can use to supplement your strength-training, interval, and ab workouts. I suggest that you do yoga moves one to three times a week—to clear your mind and stretch and work your muscles. As you get advanced with yoga moves, you can even choose a more vigorous style of yoga, like the vinyasa on page 336 or the Iron Yoga on page 343.

You can do moves at the end of a workout or as a separate session on your off days. For starters, try all of the poses once to see how they stretch your muscles, and then mix and match the poses for your workouts. During each session, aim to do four to six poses two or three times—holding each stretch for two full breaths (meaning that you inhale and exhale very slowly).

After the yoga poses, I've also included a section detailing some Pilates moves—moves that specifically work your core and will help build abdominal strength. You can substitute some of these Pilates moves, which start on page 347, for your ab workout.

WALK THIS WAY

Don't want to bring your yoga mat into your office cafeteria? Then walk it off. New research shows that you don't have to break a sweat to get mood-enhancing benefits from exercise. A brisk walk increases your heart rate, thus increasing bloodflow to your brain. That triggers the release of serotonin, the feel-good hormone that helps you feel energized and alert—not tense and stressed.

Yoga Poses

LYING DOWN LEG RAISE

Lie on your back and raise your right leg. Hold your right big toe with the first two fingers of your right hand (or hold a towel looped around your foot) and lower your leg smoothly toward your right shoulder. Go as far as you can and hold. Gently release and repeat with your left leg and hand.

SPINAL STRETCH

Sitting cross-legged, press your butt bones into the floor and lengthen your spine, reaching up with the crown of your head. You can sit on a firm pillow or folded blankets if that's more comfortable. Place your right hand on your left knee, inhale and lengthen your spine, then exhale and twist to the left. Breathe, return to the center, switch sides, and repeat. Slide your left hand onto the floor and extend your right arm overhead. Inhale and reach your fingers up toward the ceiling, then exhale and reach to the left, stretching your right side. Breathe, switch sides, and repeat, reaching to the right.

TREE

Stand with your feet rooted firmly to the floor. Keeping your left leg strong, bend your right leg and set your foot against the inside of your left thigh. Place your palms together in a prayer pose and extend your arms straight up to the ceiling. Hold, then switch legs.

FORWARD HERO

Sit on your heels, then slide your heels out to the side so your butt is touching the floor. Sit upright, inhale, and raise both arms, bringing your elbows by your ears. Keeping your butt on the floor, reach forward with your torso and drape your body over your knees.

PLOW

Lie on your back, arms at your sides and legs straight up, so your body forms a 90-degree angle. Squeeze your abs, keep your legs straight, and bring your legs back overhead. Try to touch the floor with your toes. Keep your chin away from your chest.

DOWNWARD DOG

Start on all fours with your hands shoulder-width apart and slowly lift your knees off the floor. Shift your hips as far back as possible to lengthen your spine and straighten your legs only to the extent that your spine can remain elongated. The position looks like an inverted V.

WARRIOR I

From Downward Dog, take one foot forward between your hands so that your forward thigh is parallel to the ground. Turn your back heel down and square your hips toward the front. Open up your chest by raising your arms over your head and putting your palms together. Lean your head back and lengthen your lower back by moving your tailbone toward the ground (keep your back leg straight). Hold, then switch sides.

COBBLER'S POSE

Sit down on the floor or a yoga block or blanket with the soles of your feet pressed together. (You can keep your back pressed against a wall for additional support.) Drop your knees so your inside thighs open up comfortably.

LUNGE

On all fours, step your left foot forward so your toes line up with your fingers and your knee is over your ankle. Next, slide your right leg behind you with your knee on the floor. Keep your spine long and straight and your shoulder blades down. To deepen the stretch, press your hips forward and down and your collarbones up. Breathe, switch sides, and repeat.

TRIANGLE POSE

Standing with your legs wider than shoulder-width apart, point your left toe to the side and your right foot forward. Place your left hand on your left shin or ankle, and your right hand on your right ribs. Then roll your torso open to the right so your shoulder lines up over your left shoulder. If you feel steady, lift your right arm straight up toward the ceiling so it's in line with your left arm. Keep your spine long and look up at your right arm. If this bothers your neck, gaze straight ahead. Breathe, switch sides, and repeat.

RECLINED TWIST

Lie on your back with your arms extended. Bring your knees to your chest at about a 45-degree angle. With an exhale, lower your knees to the left, keeping them stacked on top of each other. Hold, then switch sides.

CLASSIC RELAXATION

Lie on the floor with your eyes closed. Let your arms rest to your sides, with your fingers relaxed. Let your legs relax. Take 10 seconds to breathe in and 10 seconds to breathe out. Continue as long as you like.

High-Intensity Posing

IF YOU'RE INTO mat work, then you know you can get a good calorie burn from stretching, bending, and twisting. An active sequence of yoga flows—a form called vinyasa—burns more than 450 calories an hour. These two flows provide a total-body burn. Repeat each one 5 to 10 times.

FLOW 1: CHAIR POSE
TARGETS: LOWER BODY

BACKBEND
Stand with your feet hip-width apart. Lace your fingers behind you (palms facing up). Inhaling, bend from your upper back, lift your chest, and press your shoulders down.

FORWARD BEND

Soften your knees and bend forward as you exhale, letting your torso hang in front of your thighs. Keeping your arms straight and fingers locked together, lift them up and over your head (ultimately reaching toward the floor in front of your feet).

CHAIR

Inhale and bend your knees into a squat. Unlock and straighten your fingers, then separate your arms. When your thighs are nearly parallel to the floor, move your arms toward your ears. Keep your weight on your heels. Inhale, stand up, and lower your arms to your sides. Exhale.

FLOW 2: DOG POSE
TARGETS: UPPER BODY

DOWNWARD DOG

Start on all fours with your hands shoulder-width apart and slowly lift your knees off the floor. Shift your hips as far back as possible to lengthen your spine, and straighten your legs only to the extent that your spine can remain elongated. The position looks like an inverted V.

PLANK

Inhale as you shift forward into the top of a Pushup position with your arms straight. Exhale, bend your elbows (keep them pointing back and hugging your body), and lower your body until your chest is on the ground.

COBRA

Uncurl your toes so the tops of your feet are touching the ground, and press your tailbone down. Hug your elbows in as you inhale, straighten your arms (keep a slight bend), and lift your chest off the ground. Exhale as you gently release your body back to the ground. Inhale, curl your toes under, and press your hips up and back into Downward Dog. Exhale.

Buff-Body Yoga

IRON YOGA ISN'T a way to combine working out and doing chores. It's a workout that combines two popular forms of exercise into one total-body routine. Here's how it works: While you're lunging or balancing in a yoga pose, your legs and torso muscles are working hard to keep you upright. If you add a pair of dumbbells (2 to 5 pounds), suddenly your upper-body muscles are working, too, so that you get the benefits of a stronger lower body, greater flexibility, straighter posture, and reduced stress, along with stronger arms, shoulders, and back. Triathlete Anthony Carillo created Iron Yoga as a way to fit yoga into his grueling training schedule, but any level of exerciser can do the routine. If you're a yoga novice, practice the poses without weights for 2 to 4 weeks until you feel comfortable, and then add dumbbells.

CRUNCHED FOR TIME

Researchers at the University of Virginia found that it takes 250,000 crunches to burn a pound of fat. That's 100 crunches a day for 7 years. Chances are you can't wait that long. Still, in the quest for a flat stomach, you'll take an extra burn wherever you can get it, like these quick ways to burn 100 calories.

▶ Ride a stationary bike at 20 mph for 4 minutes 52 seconds.

▶ Shovel snow for 12 minutes.

▶ Walk uphill for 13 minutes.

▶ Rake leaves for 20 minutes.

▶ Give a full-body massage for 19½ minutes.

▶ Walk the dog for 23 minutes.

▶ Slow dance for 36 minutes.

▶ Tap your foot 9,351 times.

IRON YOGA POSES

CHAIR POSE WITH ROW

With your feet together and a dumbbell in each hand, sit back until your thighs are almost parallel to floor. (Beginners don't have to go so low.) Keep your back flat and look at the floor about 2 feet in front of you. Rotate your palms up and press ends of dumbbells together; don't let arms touch knees. Without moving your left arm, inhale and bend your right elbow back toward the ceiling and pull the dumbbell toward your chest. Exhale and lower. Repeat with your left arm once. Repeat with both arms at the same time and hold for one static contraction. Lower and stand up.

TREE POSE WITH PRESS AND ROTATION

Balancing on your left foot, place your right foot on the inside of your left thigh. (Beginners can place the foot on the inside of the calf or keep toes lightly touching floor.) Bring the dumbbells above your shoulders, palms facing in. Inhale and press the right dumbbell overhead, keeping your arm close to your ear. Then exhale and pull back down. Repeat with your left arm once, then with both arms at the same time, pressing the dumbbells together when overhead and holding for one static contraction. Lower and switch legs.

WARRIOR II WITH RAISE AND CURL

Step your right foot back about 4 feet. Turn your right foot out and rotate your torso to the right to square your hips and shoulders over the center of your body. Keep your left foot pointing and head looking straight ahead. Bend your left knee over your ankle until your thigh is about parallel to the floor. Raise your right arm behind you to shoulder height, palm up. Hold your left arm over your left knee, palm down. Inhale and raise the left dumbbell straight up in front to shoulder height. Exhale and lower the dumbbell. Do just once. Without moving your left arm, inhale and bend your right elbow, curling the dumbbell toward your shoulder (not shown). Exhale and press the dumbbell back to the starting position. Do just once. Raise your left arm and bend your right arm at the same time and hold for one static contraction. Return to the starting position and repeat with opposite legs and arms. Finish standing with feet together.

WARRIOR III WITH KICKBACK

Step your left foot back about 3 feet (not shown). Lean forward from your hips, bring the right dumbbell to your right armpit with elbow lifted, and raise the left dumbbell straight in front to shoulder height, palm facing in. Lift your left foot off the floor and extend your left leg straight back with toes pointed to form a straight line from left dumbbell to left toes. (Beginners can rest the extended arm on top of a chair for balance.) Inhale and extend your right arm, rotating the palm toward the ceiling, as you press the dumbbell behind you. Exhale and curl the dumbbell back toward your armpit. Do two reps, and then hold for one static contraction. Return to the starting position, lower your arms and leg, and repeat with your opposite leg raised, switching arms.

Pilates Moves

IT'S NO SECRET that staying in shape gets harder as you get older. (To prove it: In a University of Vermont study of women ages 20 to 60, researchers found that the oldest had 55 percent more belly fat than the youngest.) One of the ways to counter the effects of aging and too much potato salad is through the Abs Diet eating and exercise program. Abdominal exercises are one of the components that will help flatten and tone your stomach, but you don't have to be limited to the 50-"6-pack" of abdominal exercises I outlined earlier in the book. You can learn a lot from taking a Pilates class—a class that focuses on building and working all of the muscles in your core and torso.

One of the keys to Pilates training is to maintain what the experts call a neutral spine—that is, the position that keeps your abdominal muscles active but not too tight to allow an equal distribution of force throughout your torso. To find that position for yourself, locate a spot about 2 inches below your belly button. Now pull those muscles in and up—but not too hard. (It should feel like you're trying to squeeze into a pair of pants that's just a little too tight.) That's what a neutral spine feels like—and it's the position you should hold for all your moves. Pick four or five of these moves for the abdominal component of the Abs Workout, or just substitute one or two in your regular circuit.

Pilates Moves

SWIMMING

Lie facedown on a mat or carpeted floor with your legs extended behind you. Press your pelvis toward the floor and draw your navel toward your spine. Raise your right arm and left leg as high as comfortably possible. Lift your head and chest off the floor and begin to alternate your arms and legs in a rhythmic swimming motion, inhaling and exhaling for 10 repetitions per side.

TOE DIP

Lie on your back with your legs bent at 90 degrees—thighs straight up and calves parallel to the floor. Rest your hands at your sides, palms down. Keep your abs contracted and press your lower back toward the floor. Inhale and lower your left leg for a count of two, moving only from your hip and dipping your toes toward the floor (without letting them touch it). Exhale and raise your leg back to the starting position for a count of two. Repeat with your right leg, and continue alternating until you've done 12 reps with each leg.

SWAN LIE

Lie facedown on a mat or carpeted floor with your legs extended behind you and the tops of your feet flat on the floor. With your arms extended in front of you, hands with palms down, raise your upper body, chest, and head. Then raise your legs. Pause, then lower your upper body, followed by your legs. Repeat 10 times.

LEG CIRCLE

Lie on your back with your legs extended along the floor. Raise your left leg toward the ceiling, with toes pointed and hands at your sides, palms down. Hold for 10 to 60 seconds. Make a small circle on the ceiling with your left toes, rotating your leg from your hip. Inhale as you begin the circle and exhale as you finish. Keep your body as still as possible—no rocking—by tightening your abs. Do six circles, then reverse direction for six more. Repeat with the other leg.

CRISSCROSS

Start as in the Toe Dip but with your hands behind your head, elbows out to the sides. Curl up to raise your head, neck, and shoulders off the floor. As you inhale, rotate your torso to the right, bringing your right knee and left shoulder toward each other and extending your left leg toward the ceiling in a diagonal line from your hips. As you exhale, rotate to the left, bringing your left knee toward your right shoulder and extending your right leg. That's one repetition. Do six.

LEG KICK

Lie on your left side with your legs straight and together so your body forms one long line. Prop yourself up on your left elbow and forearm, lifting your ribs off the floor and your head toward the ceiling. Place your right hand lightly on the floor in front of you for balance. Raise your right leg to hip level and flex your foot so your toes are pointing forward. Exhale as you kick, swinging your right leg forward as far as comfortably possible and pulsing for two counts. Inhale, point your toes, and swing your leg back past your left leg. That's one rep. Do six without lowering your leg. Then switch sides and repeat.

BACK EXTENSION WITH ROTATION

Lie on your stomach with your forehead on your hands, palms on the floor.
Separate your feet to hip width. Pull your abs in. Raise your head,
shoulders, and chest off the floor. Rotate your upper body to the right and
back to center, then lower. Repeat to the left side, and continue alternating
until you've done six rotations to each side.

SHOULDER BRIDGE

Lie on your back with your knees bent, feet flat on the floor at a comfortable distance apart, heels close to your butt. Tighten your glutes and tilt your pelvis forward, raising your hips toward the ceiling slowly until your body forms a straight line from your shoulders to your knees. Keeping your hips aligned, lift your left foot off the floor and extend your leg straight out. Pause, then lower and repeat with the right leg. Then slowly lower your body back to the floor. Repeat 10 times.

GET ENERGIZED

Sometimes, our bodies need the slow, calming pace of yoga or Pilates, but sometimes, when we're feeling especially sluggish, we need to be jump-started like a dead battery—with a jolt of energy that sends us rocketing through the day. For a 5-minute energy builder that will also burn a few calories, do high-intensity moves that get your blood flowing, your muscles stretched, and your mind ready to take on the children, the clients, or the clients who act like children.

Skip hops. Step forward with your left foot and as you land, hop into the air, bending your right knee in front. Land on your right foot and hop again. Do for 2 minutes.

March. March in place as quickly as possible, letting your arms swing naturally. Do for 30 seconds.

Jump rope. Do it for 30 seconds, landing softly on the balls of your feet. No rope? Mimic the motion without one.

One-leg hop. Stand on one foot, hands on hips. Jump straight up, landing softly with a bent knee. Do 15 seconds on each leg.

The Abs Diet
Maintenance Plan

YOU'VE REACHED YOUR GOAL, AND that's reason to celebrate. But it doesn't give you license to go back to breakfasts of leftover jalapeño poppers. However, you have earned a reprieve. You've built your body to churn fat and build lean muscle. With that base, you're at the point where your body is doing a lot of the work for you. Here's a primer for maintaining the body you've built.

SUBJECT	GUIDELINE
Diet basics	You've adjusted well, and you can continue eating six meals a day by focusing on the Powerfoods—and the super ingredients, like protein, fiber, and whole-grain carbohydrates. Keep drinking smoothies regularly and adding a source of protein to every snack.
Cheating	You can up your cheating meal to a cheating day where you treat yourself to anything you want. Just keep it confined to 1 day rather than spreading it out over several meals on several days. That will increase the chances you'll stay focused and maintain good eating habits.
Exercise program	You're in maintenance mode now. Keep going with the program if you like, but you can also scale back to 1 or 2 days a week of strength training and 1 day a week of interval training. Research at the human performance laboratory at Ball State University has shown that lifters can maintain their muscle with just one workout a week.

(continued)

357

SUBJECT	GUIDELINE
Abdominal workout	Do a circuit of abdominal exercises before your strength training workouts. Move up to advanced exercises. Now that you can see your abs, you will want to increase the intensity. Still, for maximum growth, you shouldn't work your abs more than 2 or 3 days a week.

Nutritional Values of Common Foods

THE NEW TREND TOWARD LOW-carb diets has a lot of us eating plenty of fat and protein. But many of us are missing out on the valuable micronutrients found in whole grains, fruits, vegetables, and other foods that are verboten on a low-carb diet.

It might seem easier to ensure your daily value of nutrients by popping a multivitamin instead of eating a balanced diet. But there are two problems with nutrition that comes in a plastic container: First, multivitamins have no fiber, so this critical nutrient is missing if all you do is pop a pill for protection. Second, foods are loaded with plenty of nutrients beyond the standard vitamins C and E—and the importance of many of these nutrients, called phytochemicals, is only now being understood. "In a balanced diet, there are thousands of antioxidants. In pill form, you're just getting a few out of the thousands," says Edgar Miller, MD, PhD, of Johns Hopkins University in Baltimore.

To see how nutritionally complete your diet is, refer to the following chart for each food's vitamin and mineral values, and tally your total intake. If you come up short of the Recommended Dietary Allowances (RDAs) for women, don't worry. Just eat more foods high in whatever vitamins or minerals you're lacking, and take a multivitamin/mineral supplement each day.

	VITAMIN A (MCG)	VITAMIN B$_1$ (THIAMIN) (MG)	VITAMIN B$_6$ (MG)	FOLATE (MCG)	VITAMIN C (MG)
RDAS FOR WOMEN	700	1.1	1.3	400	75
Almonds (1 ounce)	0	0.05	0.03	11	0
Apple (1 medium)	8	0.02	0.06	4	6
Apricot (1)	67	0.01	0.02	3	3.50
Artichoke (1 medium)	0	0.10	0.15	87	15
Asparagus (1 medium spear)	12	0.02	0.01	8	1
Avocado (1)	122	0.20	0.60	124	16
Bacon (3 slices)	0	0.08	0.07	0.40	0
Bagel (4")	0	0.15	0.05	20	0
Banana (1 medium)	7	0.04	0.40	24	10
Beans, baked (1 cup)	13	0.40	0.34	61	8
Beans, black (1 cup cooked)	1	0.40	0.12	256	0
Beans, kidney (1 cup cooked)	0	0.28	0.21	230	2
Beans, lima (½ cup cooked)	32	0.12	0.16	22	9
Beans, navy (1 cup cooked)	0.36	0.40	0.30	255	1.64
Beans, pinto (1 cup cooked)	0	0.17	0.16	294	1.37
Beans, refried (1 cup)	0	0.07	0.36	28	15
Beans, white (1 cup cooked)	0	0.20	0.17	145	0
Beef, ground lean (3 ounces)	0	0.06	0.24	7	0
Beer (12 ounces)	0	0.02	0.18	21	0
Beets (½ cup)	3	0.02	0.05	74	3
Blueberries (1 pint)	17	0.11	0.15	17	28
Bran, wheat (1 cup)	0	0.14	0.35	14	0
Bread, rye (1 slice)	0.26	0.14	0.02	35	0.13
Bread, white (1 slice)	0	0.11	0.02	28	0
Bread, whole grain (1 slice)	0	0.11	0.10	30	0.08

VITAMIN E (MG)	CALCIUM (MG)	MAGNESIUM (MG)	POTASSIUM (MG)	SELENIUM (MCG)	ZINC (MG)	CALORIES
15	1,000	320	4,700	55	8	
6	71	86	180	0	1	170
0.25	8	7	148	0	0.06	80
0.30	5	3.50	90	0.03	0.07	20
0.24	56	77	474	0.26	0.60	25
0.18	4	2	32	0.37	0.10	5
3	22	78	1,204	0.80	0.84	250
0.06	2	6	107	12	0.70	110
0.04	16	26	90	28	1	247
0.12	6	32	422	1	0.20	110
1.35	127	81	752	12	4	239
0.14	46	120	610	2	1.90	240
0.05	62	74	717	2	1.80	260
0.12	27	63	485	1.70	0.70	229
0.73	127	107	670	11	1.90	255
1.61	72	70	495	19	1.70	245
0	88	83	675	3	3	240
1.74	161	113	1,004	2.30	2.50	249
0.15	7	19	265	0	4	185
0	18	21	89	2.50	0.04	153
0.03	11	16	221	0.50	0.24	29
1.65	17	17	223	0.30	0.50	165
0.54	26	220	426	28	3	120
0.11	23	13	53	10	0.36	83
0.06	38	6	25	4.30	0.20	67
0.09	24	14	53	8	0.30	65

	VITAMIN A (MCG)	VITAMIN B₁ (THIAMIN) (MG)	VITAMIN B₆ (MG)	FOLATE (MCG)	VITAMIN C (MG)
RDAS FOR WOMEN	700	1.1	1.3	400	75
Breakfast sandwich, fast-food (bacon, egg, and cheese)	0	0.53	0.16	73	2
Brussels sprouts (½ cup)	60	0.08	0.14	47	48
Cake, coffee (1 piece)	20	0.10	0.03	27	0.11
Cake, frosted (1 piece)	10	0.01	0.02	7	0.04
Canadian bacon (2 slices)	0	0.40	0.20	2	0
Candy, nonchocolate (1 package)	0	0	0	0	0
Cantaloupe (1 medium wedge)	345	0.04	0.07	21	37
Carrot (1)	734	0.04	0.08	12	4
Cauliflower (1 cup)	2	0.06	0.22	57	46
Celery (1 cup, strips)	55	0.03	0.10	45	4
Cereal, whole grain, with raisins (½ cup)	3	0.16	0.10	22	0.55
Cheddar cheese (1 slice)	75	0.01	0.02	5	0
Chef's salad with no dressing (1½ cups)	146	0.40	0.40	101	16
Cherries, sweet, raw (1 cup)	30	0.07	0.05	5.80	10
Chicken, skinless (½ breast)	4	0.04	0.32	2	0.71
Chickpeas (1 cup cooked)	4	0.19	0.22	282	2
Chili with beans (1 cup)	87	0.12	0.30	59	4
Chips, potato, light (1 ounce)	0	0.05	0.22	8	3.40
Chocolate (1.45 ounces)	20	0.05	0.01	5	0
Cinnamon bun (1)	0	0.12	0	17	0.06
Citrus fruits and frozen concentrate juices (12 ounces)	7	0.17	0.30	31	324
Clams, fried (¾ cup)	101	0.11	0.07	41	11.25
Coffee (1 cup)	0	0	0	5	0
Collards (1 cup cooked)	1,542	0.08	0.24	177	35

VITAMIN E (MG)	CALCIUM (MG)	MAGNESIUM (MG)	POTASSIUM (MG)	SELENIUM (MCG)	ZINC (MG)	CALORIES
15	1,000	320	4,700	55	8	
0.60	160	25	211	36.0	2	441
0.34	28	16	247	1.17	0.26	28
0.11	76	10	63	9	0.25	180
0	18	14	84	1.40	0.30	239
0.16	5	10	181	11	0.80	137
0	0	0	0	0	0	230
0.05	9	12	272	0.40	0.18	21
0.40	20	7	195	0.06	0.15	35
0.08	22	15	303	0.60	0.30	25
0.33	50	14	322	0.50	0.16	17
0.40	33	70	207	10	1	195
0.08	204	8	28	4	0.90	114
0	235	49	401	37	3	267
0.20	21	16	325	0.90	0.09	90
0.08	6.50	16	150	11	0.50	130
0.60	80	79	477	6	2.50	269
1.46	120	115	934	3	5	220
0.62	10	18	285	2	0.17	142
0.83	78	26	153	2	0.83	230
0.48	10	3.60	19	5	0.10	418
0.24	85	68	1,336	1	0.41	186
0	71	16	366	33	1.60	560
0.05	2	5	114	0	0.02	2
1.67	266	38	220	1	0.50	61

	VITAMIN A (MCG)	VITAMIN B₁ (THIAMIN) (MG)	VITAMIN B₆ (MG)	FOLATE (MCG)	VITAMIN C (MG)
RDAS FOR WOMEN	**700**	**1.1**	**1.3**	**400**	**75**
Cookie, chocolate chip (1)	0.04	0.01	0.01	0.90	0
Corn (1 cup)	0.26	0.06	0.16	115	12
Cottage cheese, low-fat (1 cup)	25	0.05	0.15	27	0
Crackers (12)	0	0.17	0	0	0
Cranberry juice cocktail (1 cup)	1	0.02	0.05	0	90
Cream cheese (1 tablespoon)	53	0	0	2	0
Cucumber with peel (½ cup)	10	0.01	0.02	7	2.76
Doughnut (1)	17	0.10	0.03	24	0.09
Egg, whole (1 large)	84	0.03	0.06	22	0
Eggplant (1 cup)	4	0.08	0.09	14	1
English muffin, whole wheat (1)	0.09	0.25	0.05	36	0
Fig bar cookies (2 bars)	3	0.05	0.02	11	0.10
Fish, white (1 fillet)	60	0.26	0.50	26	0
French fries (10)	0	0.07	0.16	8	6
Fruit, dried (1 ounce)	208	0.01	0.05	1.1	1
Fruit juice, unsweetened (1 cup)	0	0.02	0.06	35	40
Garlic (1 clove)	0	0	0.04	0.09	0.90
Graham cracker (1 large rectangular piece)	0	0.03	0.01	6	0
Granola bar (1)	2	0.06	0.02	6	0.22
Grape juice (1 cup)	1	0.07	0.16	8	0.25
Ham (1 slice)	0	0.20	0.10	1	0
Hamburger, fast-food, with condiments and vegetables (1)	4	0.30	0.12	52	2
Hot dog, fast-food (1)	0	0.44	0.09	85	0.09
Ice cream (1 serving)	6	0.03	0.04	11	0.46
Jam or preserves (1 tablespoon)	0.20	0	0	2	2

VITAMIN E (MG)	CALCIUM (MG)	MAGNESIUM (MG)	POTASSIUM (MG)	SELENIUM (MCG)	ZINC (MG)	CALORIES
15	**1,000**	**320**	**4,700**	**55**	**8**	
0.26	2.50	3	14	0	0.06	63
0.15	8	44	343	1.54	1.36	120
0.02	138	11	194	20	0.86	180
0	28	12	48	2.40	0.20	155
0	8	5	46	0	0.18	137
0.04	12	1	17	0.40	0.10	51
0	7	6	75	0	0.10	8
0.90	21	9	60	4	0.30	230
0.50	25	5	63	15	0.50	74
0.40	6	11	122	0.10	0.12	35
0.26	101	21	106	17	0.61	134
0.21	20	9	66	1	0.12	111
0.39	51	65	625	25	2	168
0.12	4	11	211	0.20	0.20	100
0.31	11.82	11.13	226	0	0.14	69
0	160	9	154	0	0.20	117
0	5	0.75	12	0.40	0	4
0.05	3	4	19	1	0.10	59
0.32	15	24	82	4	0.50	117
0	23	25	334	0.25	0.13	154
0.10	2	5	94	6	0.50	30
0.42	126	23	251	20	2	512
0.10	108	27	190	29	2	242
0	72	19	164	1.65	0.40	133
0	4	0.80	15	0.40	0	56

	VITAMIN A (MCG)	VITAMIN B₁ (THIAMIN) (MG)	VITAMIN B₆ (MG)	FOLATE (MCG)	VITAMIN C (MG)
RDAS FOR WOMEN	700	1.1	1.3	400	75
Kale (1 cup)	955	0.07	0.11	18	33
Ketchup (1 tablespoon)	7	0	0.02	2	2
Kiwifruit (1 medium)	3	0.02	0.07	19	70
Lasagna, meat (7 ounces)	61	0.19	0.20	16	12
Lentils (1 cup cooked)	4.75	0.33	0.35	358	0.22
Lettuce, iceberg (1 cup)	8	0.02	0.03	31	2
Lettuce, romaine (½ cup)	81	0.02	0.02	38	7
Liver, beef (3 ounces)	8,042	0.16	0.86	215	1.62
Lunchmeat, salami (3 slices)	0	0.10	0.08	0.34	0
Macaroni and cheese (8 ounces)	48	0.25	0	0	0
Meat loaf (1 slice)	20	0.10	0.14	12	0.62
Melon, honeydew (1 cup)	5	0.07	0.16	34	32
Milk, fat-free (1 cup)	5	0.10	0.10	12	2
Milk, soy (1 cup)	0	0.15	0.16	40	0
Muffin, blueberry (1)	13	0.10	0.01	42	0.63
Mushrooms (1 cup sliced)	0	0.09	0.10	12	2
Nachos with cheese (6–8)	170	0.20	0.20	12	1
Nectarine (1)	23	0.05	0.03	7	7
Oatmeal (1 cup)	0.12	0.12	0.10	13	0
Olives (1 tablespoon)	1.70	0	0	0	0
Onion rings (10 medium)	0.98	0.10	0.07	64	0.68
Oyster (1 medium)	4.20	0.01	0.01	1.40	0.52
Pancakes (2)	7.60	0.16	0.07	28	0.15
Pasta with red sauce (4.5 ounces)	0	0.13	0.10	4	6
Peach (1 medium)	16	0.02	0.02	4	6
Peanut butter (2 tablespoons)	0	0.03	0.15	24	0
Peanuts (1 ounce)	0	0.12	0.07	41	0

VITAMIN E (MG)	CALCIUM (MG)	MAGNESIUM (MG)	POTASSIUM (MG)	SELENIUM (MCG)	ZINC (MG)	CALORIES
15	1,000	320	4,700	55	8	
1	180	23	417	1.17	0.23	39
0.20	3	3	57	0.04	0	15
1	26	13	237	0.15	0.10	50
0.94	220	41	372	28	3	318
2.97	37	71	731	5.54	2.51	230
0.02	11	4	84	0.28	0.10	8
0.04	9	4	69	0.10	0.06	5
0.43	5	18	300	31	4.50	162
0.05	1.34	2.86	63	4	0.54	150
0	102	0	111	0	0	415
0.10	43	22	295	0	4	231
0.04	11	18	403	1.24	0.16	61
0.10	301	27	406	5	1	83
0	80	60	440	3	0.90	100
0.47	32	9	70	6	0.30	158
0.10	5	10	355	8	0.70	15
0	311	63	196	18	?	296
1	8	12	273	0	0.23	70
0.26	19	51	175	0	1.43	150
0.14	7	0.30	0.67	0.08	0	10
0.39	86	19	152	3	0.41	370
0.12	6	7	22	9	13	41
0.65	96	15	133	10	0.30	173
1.40	41	13	207	11	0.66	216
0.70	6	9	186	0.10	0.17	70
0	12	51	214	2	1	190
2	15	50	186	2	1	165

	VITAMIN A (MCG)	VITAMIN B₁ (THIAMIN) (MG)	VITAMIN B₆ (MG)	FOLATE (MCG)	VITAMIN C (MG)
RDAS FOR WOMEN	**700**	**1.1**	**1.3**	**400**	**75**
Pear (1 medium)	1.60	0.02	0.05	12	7
Pepper, chile, raw (½ pepper)	21.6	0.03	0.23	10.35	65
Peppers, sweet (10 strips)	78	0.04	0.13	13	70
Pie, apple (1 piece)	37	0.03	0.04	32	4
Pizza, cheese (1 slice)	74	0.20	0.04	35	1
Pizza, vegetable (1 slice)	58	0.40	0.50	116	79
Plum (1)	21	0.03	0.05	1.45	6
Popcorn (1 cup)	0.80	0.02	0.02	2	0
Pork (3 ounces)	0	0.80	0.30	3	0
Potatoes, mashed (1 cup)	8.40	0.20	0.50	17	13
Potato salad (1 cup)	2.93	0.20	0.40	19	19
Potpie, chicken	256	0.30	0.20	41	2
Pretzels (10 twists)	0	0.30	0.07	103	0
Raisins (1.5 ounces)	0	0.05	0.08	1.28	2.30
Raspberries (10)	0.38	0.01	0.01	4	5
Rice, brown (1 cup)	0	0.20	0.30	8	0
Rice, white (1 cup)	0	0.03	0.15	5	0
Ricotta cheese, part skim (½ cup)	132	0.03	0.02	16	0
Salad dressing, light Italian (1 tablespoon)	0	0	0	0	0
Salmon (3 ounces)	9.84	0.20	0.71	22	0
Salsa (½ cup)	44	0.05	0.16	21	18
Sauerkraut (1 cup)	1.42	0.03	0.18	34	21
Sausage (1 link)	0	0.05	0.01	0.26	0
Shrimp (4 large)	0	0.01	0.03	0.77	0.48
Soft drink with caffeine (12 ounces)	0	0	0	0	0
Soup, cream of chicken (1 cup)	179	0.07	0.07	7	1.24

VITAMIN E (MG)	CALCIUM (MG)	MAGNESIUM (MG)	POTASSIUM (MG)	SELENIUM (MCG)	ZINC (MG)	CALORIES
15	1,000	320	4,700	55	8	
0.20	15	12	198	0.17	0.17	100
0.30	6	10	145	0.20	0.12	2
0.36	7	6.46	105	0	0	5
1.78	13	8	76	1	0.20	296
0	117	16	113	13	1	272
2	189	65	548	23	2	170
0	3	5	114	0.30	0.07	40
0	1	11	24	0.80	0.30	31
0.20	6	15	253	14	2	191
0.04	46	38	621	2	0.60	201
0.14	14	36	551	10	0.60	358
4	33	24	256	0.70	1	484
0.21	22	21	88	3	0.50	229
0.30	12	13	350	0.26	0.08	127
0.17	5	4	28	0.04	0.08	10
0.06	20	84	84	19	1	216
0.06	16	19	55	12	0.80	205
0.09	337	19	155	21	1.70	171
0	0	0	2	0.20	0	26
0.95	11	28	475	35	0.60	175
1.53	39	17	275	0.50	0.30	41
0.14	43	18	241	0.90	0.30	45
0.03	1.30	1.56	25	1.87	0.24	125
0	9	7	40	9	0.30	22
0	10	3	3	0.34	0	154
0.25	181	17	272	8	0.67	225

	VITAMIN A (MCG)	VITAMIN B₁ (THIAMIN) (MG)	VITAMIN B₆ (MG)	FOLATE (MCG)	VITAMIN C (MG)
RDAS FOR WOMEN	**700**	**1.1**	**1.3**	**400**	**75**
Soup, tomato (1 cup)	29.28	0.09	0.11	15	66
Soybeans (1 cup cooked)	14	0.47	0.10	200	31
Spaghetti with meatballs (1½ cups)	46	0.38	0.43	101	24
Spareribs (3 ounces)	1.91	0.26	0.22	3	0
Spinach (1 cup)	140	0.02	0.06	58	8
Steak (different cuts)	0	0.10	0.30	6	0
Strawberries (1 cup)	1.66	0.03	0.09	40	97
Submarine sandwich	71	1	0.10	87	12
Sunflower seeds (¼ cup)	5	0	0.28	82	0.50
Sweet potato (1)	350	0.09	0.25	9	19
Taco salad (1.5 cups)	71	0.10	0.20	83	4
Toaster pastry (1)	148	0.20	0.20	15	0
Tofu (4 ounces)	4.96	0.10	0.06	19	0
Tomato (1 medium)	26	0.02	0.05	9	8
Tuna salad (1 cup)	49	0.06	0.17	16	5
Turkey, skinless (½ breast)	0	0.16	2.26	31	0
Vegetable juice (1 cup)	188	0.10	0.30	51	67
Walnuts (1 cup)	37	0.27	0.70	82	4
Watermelon (1 wedge)	104	0.20	0.40	6	31
Wheat germ (½ cup)	0	0.20	0.40	81	0
Whey protein powder (2 teaspoons)	0	0	0	0	0
Wine, red (3.5 ounces)	0	0	0.03	2	0
Wine, white (3.5 ounces)	0	0	0.01	0	0
Yogurt, low-fat (8 ounces)	2	0.10	0.09	24	1.70

VITAMIN E (MG)	CALCIUM (MG)	MAGNESIUM (MG)	POTASSIUM (MG)	SELENIUM (MCG)	ZINC (MG)	CALORIES
15	1,000	320	4,700	55	8	
2	12	7	263	0.50	0.24	180
0.02	261	108	970	3	1.64	298
4	138	66	718	39	5	545
0.20	30	15	204	24	3	338
0.60	30	24	167	0.30	0.16	10
0.11	4	19	250	12	3.26	217
0.50	27	22	253	1	0.20	46
0	189	60	394	31	2.60	386
12	42	127	248	21.42	1.82	205
1.42	41	27	348	0.30	0.30	103
192	51	416	4	3	0	279
0.90	17	12	57	6.30	0.30	204
0.01	434	37	150	11	1	75
0.33	6	7	146	0	0.11	35
2	35	39	365	84	1	383
0.30	39	109	1,142	95	5	413
12	26	27	467	1	0.50	50
0	73	253	655	21	4.28	654
0.40	41	31	479	0.30	0.20	86
0	27	275	166	91	14	104
0	0	0	260	0	0	21
0	8	13	111	0.20	0.10	88
0	9	10	80	0.20	0.07	86
0	415	37	497	11	1.88	193

Glycemic Loads for Selected Foods

Peanuts	1	Kidney beans, canned	9
Low-fat yogurt, artificially sweetened	2	Lentil soup	9
		Oatmeal cookies	9
Carrots	3	Sweet corn	9
Grapefruit	3	American rye bread	10
Green peas	3	Cheese tortellini	10
Fat-free milk	4	Frozen waffles	10
Pear	4	Honey	10
Watermelon	4	Lima beans, frozen	10
Beets	5	Low-fat yogurt, sweetened with sugar	10
Orange	5		
Peach	5	Pinto beans	10
Plum	5	White bread	10
Apple	6	Bran Chex cereal	11
Kiwifruit	6	Apple juice	12
Tomato soup	6	Banana	12
Baked beans	7	Kaiser roll	12
Chickpeas, canned	7	Orange juice	12
Grapes	7	Saltine crackers	12
Pineapple	7	Bran flakes	13
Whole-wheat bread	7	Oatmeal	13
Popcorn	8	Graham crackers	14
Soy milk	8	Special K cereal	14
Taco shells	8	Vanilla wafers	14
All-Bran cereal	9	Bran muffin	15
Grapefruit juice	9	Cheerios cereal	15
Hamburger bun	9	French bread	15

Grape-Nuts cereal	15	Angel food cake	19
Mashed potatoes	15	Cornflakes cereal	21
Shredded wheat cereal	15	French fries	22
Bread stuffing mix	16	Jelly beans	22
Cheese pizza	16	Macaroni	22
Whole-wheat spaghetti	16	Rice Krispies cereal	22
Black bean soup	17	Couscous	23
Blueberry muffin	17	Linguine	23
Corn chips	17	Long-grain rice	23
Doughnut	17	White rice	23
Grape-Nuts Flakes cereal	17	Bagel	25
Instant oatmeal	17	Baked potato	26
Rice cakes	17	Spaghetti	27
Sweet potato	17	Raisins	28
Total cereal	17	Macaroni and cheese	32
Brown rice	18	Instant rice	36
Fettuccine	18		

Index

Boldface page references indicate photographs. Underscored references indicate boxed text.